Personality Disorder

Personality Disorder

From Evidence to Understanding

Peter Tyrer
Consultant in Transformation Psychiatry, Lincolnshire Partnership NHS Foundation Trust and Emeritus Professor of Community Psychiatry, Imperial College, London

Roger Mulder
University of Otago, Christchurch

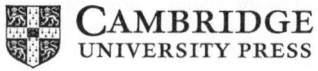

CAMBRIDGE
UNIVERSITY PRESS

University Printing House, Cambridge CB2 8BS, United Kingdom

One Liberty Plaza, 20th Floor, New York, NY 10006, USA

477 Williamstown Road, Port Melbourne, VIC 3207, Australia

314–321, 3rd Floor, Plot 3, Splendor Forum, Jasola District Centre, New Delhi – 110025, India

103 Penang Road, #05–06/07, Visioncrest Commercial, Singapore 238467

Cambridge University Press is part of the University of Cambridge.

It furthers the University's mission by disseminating knowledge in the pursuit of
education, learning, and research at the highest international levels of excellence.

www.cambridge.org
Information on this title: www.cambridge.org/9781108948371
DOI: 10.1017/9781108951685

© Royal College of Psychiatrists 2022

First published 2022

A catalogue record for this publication is available from the British Library.

Library of Congress Cataloging-in-Publication Data
Names: Tyrer, Peter J. author. | Mulder, Roger, author. | Royal College of Psychiatrists, issuing body.
Title: Personality disorder : from evidence to understanding / Peter Tyrer, Roger Mulder.
Description: Cambridge, United Kingdom ; New York, NY : Cambridge University Press, 2022. | Includes
bibliographical references and index.
Identifiers: LCCN 2021030312 (print) | LCCN 2021030313 (ebook) | ISBN 9781108948371 (paperback) |
ISBN 9781108951685 (ebook)
Subjects: MESH: Personality Disorders
Classification: LCC RC473.P56 (print) | LCC RC473.P56 (ebook) | NLM WM 190 | DDC 616.85/81–dc23
LC record available at https://lccn.loc.gov/2021030312
LC ebook record available at https://lccn.loc.gov/2021030313

ISBN 978-1-108-94837-1 Paperback

Dedicated to all those with personality disorder who have yet to be acknowledged

Contents

Contents

Foreword

When asked about those we love, we are likely to describe admirable aspects of their personality (or temperament and character). When describing those we hate, we are likely to describe defects in their personality. In routine domestic or work settings, discussion of persons tends to involve a combination of physical characteristics, present mental state and ... their characteristic personality traits. When I asked young people in two Youth Offending Teams what characteristics they sought, 'fit', 'cool' and 'good sense of humour' emerged, for boys and girls.

The impetus for this book was the International Classification of Diseases (ICD), whose recent revision 'ICD-11' needed to shed light on disorders of personality in a way that actually helped professionals working in many settings and languages and to recognise and address these conditions. Peter Tyrer and Roger Mulder, the authors of the present volume, were part of the international team making these revisions for the World Health Organization.

The nineteenth century saw the beginnings of formal diagnostic systems for mental health care in hospital populations, and also new health systems for non-clinical settings such as schools, the military or prisons. The ancient Greeks had developed systems for classifying the world around them, including its people – our modern concept 'typology' derives from two Greek words (tupos + logos), first combined in English around 1845. As an undergraduate, Charles Darwin (1809–82) displayed skill in classification of rocks that led his geology professor to choose him for the *Beagle* expedition in 1831. During that voyage his classification skills developed in biology and anthropology. In subsequent decades, several academic disciplines attempted to explore specific aspects of personality, including psychology, anthropology, criminology, philosophy and education. Medical practice generated the broad territory of 'psychopathology', within whose diagnoses some patients were described in terms of *disorder* (i.e. an abnormality) of personality. The Victorian era was also a time of charting and measuring, for example at a time when some patients in asylums were encouraged to undertake physical activity, tracking gentlemen's cricket scores might be used to measure the progress of their treatment. In the nineteenth century, there were many unhelpful avenues explored, such as the physical anthropology of 'criminality' or the genetics of moral 'degeneracy', but the early twentieth century saw measurement applied more productively in areas like occupational psychology and education. At the beginning of that century, the Vienna Psychoanalytic Society was the fulcrum of debate on mental health. Impaired social functioning is a characteristic of personality disorders. The Viennese doctor Alfred Adler (1870–1937) was particularly interested in 'character' and its shaping in childhood, first through relationships across all family members and then in community relationships. Like the authors of this book, Adler was optimistic that much suffering could be prevented, with *early* interventions during an individual's lifecourse, but we have yet to learn if this can indeed be achieved.

The horrific slaughter of the 1914–18 war saw an unprecedented, monstrous 'natural experiment' in term of medical classification. Among the wounded, the observational skills of Henry Head (1861–1940) and William Rivers (1864–1922) began a pioneering synthesis of trauma (both physical and psychological), neuroscience, social anthropology, language and psychotherapeutics. For their patients, changes in personality were notable (e.g. pre-war, in the crisis of war and post-war). However, for a hundred years, the usefulness of *evidence* based on even huge clinical case series has proved limited. Today, we have two much more potent methods to use: experimental medicine (clinical trials) and population science (epidemiology).

Today, the ICD-11 classification also gives opportunity for new research and the design and evaluation of innovative services that are grounded in research evidence. Central to the ICD approach is that it is informed by statistical science and includes 'related health problems': this is helpful when caring for patients with complex histories who are distressed (and sometimes distressing). Not only do health statistics link people in different services, they provide a common language for international collaboration. For example, in my own experience such linkages were vital in planning a mother-and-baby service for socially isolated women dependent on heroin with a long history of overdosing, contact with both social services and the criminal justice system, and limited understanding of parenting. In that hospital, the mother I remember best also had the related health problem of AIDS.

Years ago, I felt very proud when the Institute of Psychiatry made me an honorary lecturer, but most of my teaching has been in primary health care. Participants included general practitioners (GPs), school nurses, prison medical officers, occupational therapists and public health specialists. GPs see most of the patients with mental disorders, but unlike the 'common' illnesses that present in primary care (depression, anxiety or mixed anxiety and depression), there is no evidence-based pill for personality that they can offer as a first-line treatment. Using the ideas developed by Michael Balint (1896–1970), the first-line 'treatment' is usually the personality and understanding of the practitioner.

Many people working in primary care have been unwilling to apply diagnostic 'labels' to their patients with mental health needs. In this book, Tyrer and Mulder explore many reasons why psychiatrists may have been reluctant to use the term personality disorder with their patients at all. I gained some related insight while teaching GPs about the ICD-10PHC diagnoses. ICD-10PHC had printed guidelines on two sides of plastic cards: one for diagnosis and one for management of each condition. I was working then for a world-renowned professor who liked to start each seminar before handing over to me to finish up the routine bits. When the GPs asked him for authoritative advice about patients with personality disorders, he told them not to bother, 'because there was nothing they could do for them'. It seems that therapeutic pessimism can stifle engagement with these patients and Tyrer and Mulder want to change our attitudes here. In a very different setting, I was gathering data from all the 'customers' of a Job Centre Plus, including the use of the Standardised Assessment of Personality – Abbreviated Scale (SAPAS) screening question-naire (see Chapter 10 of this book). We also questioned the employment advisors about those who had completed the SAPAS. The most common response of the advisors when finding that the 'customer' had problems related to their personality was: 'hopeless'.

Before the discovery of antibiotics, therapeutic pessimism was common in patients with sexually transmitted infections. To be able to witness some improvement in the lives of service users makes a big difference for any therapeutic alliance. In my lifetime, the two most common labels for personality disorders have been antisocial and borderline, and I remember when the National Health Service would fund a few residential patients in therapeutic communities (TCs). For patients with very long-term, pervasive problems, I witnessed clear improvements in two TCs (one with mainly 'antisocial' residents and one with mainly 'borderline' residents). Individuals typically had multiple problems affecting their social functioning, such as 'complex' post-traumatic stress disorder after prolonged childhood sexual abuse or chronic dependence on alcohol. Nonetheless, over months, social functioning gradually improved and objective measures of behaviour such as attendance at accident and emergency services or police contacts changed substantially. Sadly, changes in NHS funding streams saw both those TCs close. I am on a steering group for a project about self-harm in prisons, and until the current Coronavirus pandemic my impression from psychologists in that setting was they were beginning to see some reduction in both self-harm and offending . . . I am holding my breath to see if that is maintained when the pandemic abates. The population for whom I am most optimistic was the one I saw in the first Youth Offending Teams, courtesy of funding from the charity Barnardo's. In adolescence, we could sometimes observe a real change in their trajectory over a few months, using various creative arts with groups of young people. However, that young population rarely had thorough assessments: this is where a clear, practical system like the ICD-11 could open doors to early treatment and lasting change.

In what way is ICD-11 more practical than older systems? Clinically or epidemiologically, it is clear the categorical labels of the past are no longer of value. Peter Tyrer himself led a challenge to the totally impractical terminology of 'dangerous and severe personality disorders'. A label like that practically guarantees social stigma and increased health inequalities when such people are predictably excluded from services. Across all types of people in the ICD-11 system, the severity of personality disorder is measured by the complexity of a person's problems. Patients whose functioning is significantly impaired (personality disorder) are distinguished from the much larger number with Personality difficulties – this awareness of a personality spectrum is vital to develop appropriate public health responses. Classification matters – no one likes to be called 'fat' – but a spectrum of adiposity from underweight to overweight is helpful in describing populations and morbid obesity should ring clinical alarm bells.

Thus a key message in this book is to 'embrace the personality spectrum'. To promote understanding, the World Health Organization has chosen 25th May as International Personality Spectra Day. Please note and celebrate it.

Here in the UK, the Government is in the process of reforming the Mental Health Act. This reform is long overdue, to ensure the rights of service users, appropriate training for mental health professionals and resources to provide care for people whose needs are not being met at present. A key driver of change is the NHS Long Term Plan, which commits to expanding services 'delivered through new models of integrated primary, community and social care'. Crucially the wording of this should be remembered by all:

> The new models will incorporate care for people with eating disorders, mental health rehabilitation needs and those with a diagnosis of a 'personality disorder', among other groups.

Woody Caan
Professorial Fellow, Royal Society for Public Health

Acknowledgements

This book is written at a time when developments in the science and understanding of personality disorder need as wide a distribution as possible. We therefore have tried to be fair and reasonable in discussing many areas that are contentious. The following colleagues have helped greatly in this task; if we have failed to convince the readership we take responsibility, but in part this responsibility is collective, as we have consulted widely on the more contentious topics. In particular we thank Jo Ramsden, Sharon Prince, Linda Gask and John Gunn for their help in discussing stigma; Essi Viding for helping to put psychopathy in its rightful place; Jane Cannon, Ian Gould, Elena Garralda, Jovanka Tolmac and David Skuse for helping in the placement of personality problems in children; and George Stein for clarifying personality disorder in the Old Testament. Paul Salkovskis and Michael Parsonage were very helpful in the interpretation of recent documents from the British Psychological Society, and Giles Newton-Howes and Michael Crawford gave incisive feedback. John Eagles and Louise Doughty need to be thanked for helping to promote the concept of personality difficulty in *Starting to Shrink* and *Apple Tree Yard*; Mary McMurran and Conor Duggan for being so transparent about their research; Paul Moran and Youl-Ri Kim for help in disseminating practice; Donald Black for reminding us that all is not rosy with some personality problems; Paul Emmelkamp and Katharine Meyerbröker for material assistance; Eva Burns-Lundgren, Steve Pearce, Rex Haigh and Kate Davidson for helping to crystallise the essentials of key treatments; and Jed Boardman and Catherine Gardiner for pointing out the important aspects of social prescribing. Bo Bach also provided clinical and treatment insights, John Horwood useful statistical advice and Frances Carter gave constant support and feedback. We also are very grateful to Bridget Kinnersley for her sterling work in reframing diagrams and checking the references with such care.

This book would not have been written if the ICD-11 Revision Group for the Classification of Personality Disorders had not been able to complete its work successfully. We thank the other members of the group, Roger Blashfield (USA), Lee Anna Clark (USA), Alireza Farnam (Iran), Andrea Fossati (Italy), Youl-Ri Kim (Korea), Nestor Koldobsky (Argentina), Dušica Lečíc-Toševski (Serbia), David Ndetei (Kenya), Michaela Swales (Wales) and Geoffrey Reed (WHO) for making our work so harmonious.

History of Personality and Its Disorders

Historical chapters in scientific books are generally dull even though they do not intend to be. There is an understandable need to record what happened in the past even though it may be quite irrelevant to what is going on today. We are frequently asked to remember George Santayana's comment, made by many others, that 'those who cannot remember the past are condemned to repeat it' (Santayana, 1905). But this is hardly relevant for a textbook on The Wheel. Those who concentrate on wheel technology are not going to be particularly interested, except in a voyeuristic sense, in how Neolithic people might have been able to move large blocks of stone to Stonehenge for hundreds of miles using primitive garden rollers. But with personality disorder it is different. Without some knowledge of the history of personality disorder current descriptions cannot be placed in any sort of context.

This chapter highlights the split between the general notion of personality as a universal characteristic, a safe and acceptable subject, and the more focused history of personality disorder as a psychiatric condition, a highly stigmatised subject. We can divide this history into four ages.

1.1 Age 1. The Age of Discovery (460 BC–AD 1700)

Personality as a concept has been present almost since the dawn of civilisation. It is part of the mix that makes us human. All the primates are social animals and so personality is integral to their functioning, and as humankind has become more organised in its social structures the importance of personality has correspondingly increased. Nomenclature has changed from discussion of the four humours to categories and other groupings but personality has never lost its central importance.

Hippocrates (460 BC) begins the historical story; he often does. The importance of personality comes out in his teaching of the four humours. Essentially this presents the body as a combination of four substances (or humours): black bile, yellow bile, blood and phlegm. In order for a person to stay healthy, these humours have to be in balance. Sickness is the consequence when this balance is lost. It is easy to see how this view was created, as in most illnesses there are changes in the emanations of the body that are abnormal. The correct treatment of illness was to put these humours back into balance.

But it was his disciple, Galen, a Greek who, 500 years later, served as physician to many of the Roman emperors, who attached the humours to personality. Galen was impatient to apply the work of Hippocrates to medical practice, and in his work derived the first proper classification of personality types that has persisted in various forms to the present day. So personality became attached, almost indelibly, to the four humours:

- Black bile – melancholia and depressive personality

- Yellow bile – choleric personality with aggressive and explosive outbursts
- Blood – positive forceful (sanguine) personalities with great drive
- Phlegm – passive (negative) detached personalities.

It is easy to see how three of these could subsequently be attached to personality disorder. Don't worry – they were. This was too good an idea to fade into obscurity.

Another initiator of the notion of personality types was Aristotle's pupil Theophrastus, born in 371 BC. Theophrastus was a good observer, and he begins his description of each of his personality types (which he calls 'characters') with a brief account of the person concerned, followed by their personality foibles. In all he describes 30 characters, some of which when combined resemble modern descriptions of personality types, but others demonstrate only too well that they are poor ways of grouping people.

Theophrastus is bright and inquisitive and also very nosy (a useful quality in those who want to know more about personality), and starts off with the penetrating question about diversity: 'why it is that, while all Greece lies under the same sky and all the Greeks are educated alike, it has befallen us to have characters so variously constituted?' (Theophrastus, 1909). He then describes 30 of these characters in such a way that it constitutes a prototypical classification – descriptions that the reader can pigeonhole and recognise immediately. One of the best examples is the account of the 'distrustful man' who in many ways resembles the paranoid category of the International Classification of Diseases 10 (ICD-10) and the Diagnostic and Statistical Manual of Mental Disorders (DSM) IV.

> The distrustful man is one who, having sent his slave to market, will send another to ascertain what price he gave. He will carry his money himself, and sit down every two-hundred yards to count it.
>
> (Theophrastus, 1909)

Similarly, the 'superstitious man' reflects some of the features of what is now called schizotypal personality, appearing to exhibit 'cowardice towards divine power'. Even when the soothsayer tells him that the mouse hole in his sack has no mystic significance and should be repaired by an ordinary cobbler, he proceeds to offer a sacrifice in expiation.

But then Theophrastus gets diverted into descriptions of his own personal prejudices. We read about the 'Ironical man', the 'Garrulous and the Chatty man' (obviously overlapping), the 'Gross man' (not gross in size but insensitive in behaviour), the 'Officious man' (one steeped in conventional authority) and the 'Late-learner' (one who engages in activities when too old), and it does not take much reflection to realise that these are not useful universal concepts. The 'Man of Petty Ambition' and the 'Boastful man' (an habitual liar who 'stands in the bazaar talking to foreigners of the great sums which he has at sea; about the vastness of his money-lending business and the extent of his personal gains and losses') can seem more accurate descriptions, but the 'Oligarch' (who loves authority and is covetous, not of gain, but of power), the 'Patron of Rascals' (who likes the company of those involved in 'criminal causes') and the 'Avaricious man' (who has 'excessive desire of base gain') are all obviously recognisable but not necessarily linked to personality pathology (Aldington, 1924).

These descriptions make amusing reading (see www.eudaemonist.com/biblion/charac ters), but their main interest is to show that the gossip in the Athenian marketplace of 2500 years ago is little different from the gossip of boardrooms, production lines and offices of today. We all like to gossip about others' personalities, usually sotto voce with selected people. It gives us a little thrill and puts us into special coteries of understanding. Despite the curious paradox of modern science largely ignoring disorders of personality and valiant attempts of others to suppress the term altogether, it is always with us.

George Stein has made an exhaustive and penetrating study of the psychiatric aspects of the writings revealed in the Old Testament of the Bible (Stein, 2018). The book of Proverbs (800–500 BC) is a guide to success in leading a contented and moral life. It is expressed as a series of teachings in the form of proverbs from fathers to their sons on how to achieve wisdom in life. The opposite of wisdom is folly, and the text describes a number of different fools who should not be emulated and should be avoided at all costs. The word fool in the English is a translation for several different character types found in the Hebrew text, and although these are described as bad characters, it is not difficult to detect that the 'bad character' types show many of the known features of modern day personality disorders, especially antisocial personality disorder (Stein, 2018, p. 386).

One character in particular chimes with personality disorder; the *Belial* or Scoundrel, who is described as having a perverted mind, devises evil schemes and goes around sowing discord. He is haughty and lies and spreads strife. He testifies falsely, sows discord in his family and he sounds just like a textbook example of an aggressive psychopath (Stein, 2018, p. 437). There are several other malevolent characters described in this text: the *pithy* combines antisocial behaviours with stupidity; the *ceil* is an immoral fool and is also not very bright but not as stupid as the *pithy*; the *'ewil* is an immoral antisocial type but of normal or above average intelligence; the *les* is a narcissist with arrogance and contempt for others and is also an antisocial person but of normal intelligence. The book of Proverbs also has verses which contain 21 out of the 22 antisocial character traits that comprise the Hare Psychopathy Check List (PCL-R) (see Chapter 2). The only trait that cannot be located is 'parasitic existence', but this is hardly surprising as there were few opportunities to be parasitic in society in ancient Israel.

Finally, unusual females are described in the book of Proverbs, the *essa zarah,* or the strange women, often mistranslated in English Bibles as 'the loose women'. Each of these has seductive speech, is adulterous and can dress up like a prostitute. They are loud and wayward, have itchy feet and lack any sense of identity. They can also be bitter and angry and are emotionally unstable. Stein suggests this description shows some resemblance to current Cluster B personality disorders, particularly borderline and histrionic disorder, and fulfils diagnostic criteria for both. It is quite possible that Kurt Schneider had read about these before deciding to make his own assessments of personality disorder with the prostitutes in Hamburg (see 1.3, Age 3. The Age of Investigation and Intervention).

Some would argue that it is too much of a leap into the dark to equate an immoral character of the Bible, from a rural society of the first millennium BC, with a twenty-first-century Western medical category such as a personality disorder. But the language of personality crosses millennia and cannot easily be ignored.

But although Stein equates this with psychopathy and antisocial personality disorder, the descriptions in Proverbs are basically no different from those of Theophrastus. They are character descriptions of personality and not defined in terms that naturally allow conversion to descriptions of disorder.

But these examples illustrate that personality types (i.e. descriptions of dominant features of personality) have been well described for centuries. Robert Burton, in his comprehensive account of depression and associated disorders, *The Anatomy of*

Melancholy, describes the typical melancholic as having 'a calm, quiet and patient personality' (Burton, 1621; republished 1927).

1.2 Age 2. The Age of Personality as a Substrate (1750–1950)

This title may seem odd to modern readers. But in the eighteenth and nineteenth centuries, personality and its disorder was seen as an underlying substrate to all mental illness. It is common to refer to James Prichard (1837) as a key definer of personality disorder in his description of moral insanity, but his descriptions are more those of mood (hypomania) rather than personality disorder. The same applies to Philippe Pinel's description of 'manie sans délire' (Pinel, 1809), often wrongly referred to as a description of personality pathology. 'Manie', at the time of Pinel, referred to almost all serious mental illness and did not embrace personality.

What was happening around this time was the recognition that personality problems were somewhat separate from mental illness but could also influence them. Henry Maudsley described people who would now be regarded as unequivocally antisocial:

> They display no trace of affection for their parents, or of feelings for others; the only care they evince is to contrive the means of indulging their passions and vicious propensities.
>
> (Maudsley, 1868, p. 329)

Bénédict Morel was born in Vienna but practised all his life in France, and he created a classification system that included the notion of hereditary insanity – that some individuals had congenitally nervous temperaments that made them more prone to insanity (Morel, 1852). This notion of hereditary disposition in personality disorder was a pernicious one and has persisted unfairly. It was followed by the notion of 'psychopathic inferiorities' introduced by Julius Koch in 1888, who summarised the condition as some having it from birth, some acquiring the condition and the worst group showing degenerative features (Shorter, 2005, p. 213). This was when stigma developed in earnest.

But the notion of personality as an underlying substrate influencing or creating predisposition to mental illness had taken root. Here we had a condition that was on the fringe of mental illness but could not be ignored as at the time it could prod you unwillingly into the realm of other mental disorders.

In the early twentieth century four figures dominated the study of personality: Sigmund Freud, Adolf Meyer, David Henderson and Gordon Allport. Freud's description of oral, anal and phallic phases of sexual development are too well known to go into detail here, but his description of what happens when these phases are arrested brought him into discussion of underlying personality (although he described this as character rather than personality) (Freud, 1916; republished 1963). This had a major influence on psychiatric thinking. Adolf Meyer is much less known nowadays, although he was at least is as well known as Freud in the early years of the twentieth century (Meyer, 1950). He was a German-speaking Swiss who emigrated to the USA at an early age and quickly made a name for himself as an all-round psychiatrist with an eclectic view of the subject. He accepted that psychoanalysis had something to offer but rejected its theory-based approach and much preferred one based on common sense. Unfortunately, despite being an excellent teacher, his writings are almost impossible to follow, and none of them are really quotable.

This is unfortunate because there is much that can be learned from Adolf Meyer's approach. He regarded the personality of a person as integral to the manifestation of mental illness. Put simply, something Meyer seemed incapable of doing, except in lectures, the personality of a person is the foremost mental feature and any subsequent illness was regarded as a reaction to this. This led to a somewhat confusing idea of diagnosis in which each psychiatric diagnosis, now regarded as a disorder, was described as a 'reaction type'. For the average psychiatrist this was confusing, but in making a psychiatric assessment Meyer emphasised the importance of getting to know each aspect of that person's life, their thinking and their goals. In teaching medical students, he asked each of them to assess a colleague's personality in this way in order to get what would now be described as 'whole person thinking'. He was especially concerned about a diagnostic label being given to a patient prematurely as this would inhibit further enquiry and thought. He would certainly have reinforced the concerns about over-diagnosis in psychiatry, perhaps best expressed by Allen Frances (2013), and might well have agreed that DSM really stood for 'Diagnosis for Simple Minds' (Tyrer, 2012).

The reason why Meyer became the most important figure in US psychiatry was because he bridged the different disciplines and theories swirling around the subject at the beginning of the twentieth century. He accepted the principles of psychoanalysis but felt they were overstated; he felt psychiatry should be linked to medicine but not absorbed into it, and he was very supportive of a multidisciplinary approach to treatment (his wife was a social worker).

Adolf Meyer inspired others, including Rolv Gjessing in Norway (who identified the cause of periodic catatonia) and David Henderson in Edinburgh. (Gjessing had a notice on his office door 'In the long run it all depends on personality'.) Henderson worked with Adolf Meyer early in his career and subsequently became one of the foremost psychiatrists in the United Kingdom, writing the standard textbook on the subject in 1927 (Henderson and Gillespie, 1927), with revised editions until 1961. He too referred to reaction types throughout these books, but he also developed Meyer's interest in personality further.

He published a book, *Psychopathic States* (Henderson, 1939), in which he defined three types of psychopaths. The first, equivalent to what is now commonly known as psychopathic personality was aggressive and dangerous. The second was the inadequate psychopath, a person who lived off society by swindling and cheating, was frequently in prison for minor offences, but who was not violent, and the third group, the most controversial, being eccentric people who went against social norms. He included individuals such as Lawrence of Arabia in this group, but most would not consider many of these examples to be psychopathic in the same way as the other two groups. His book was a major influence in the UK in the mid-twentieth century, and his advocacy of psychopathy as an important condition for psychiatrists to recognise led to the first hospital to treat this condition in the form of a therapeutic community. It was named the Henderson Hospital.

Gordon Allport added much more rigour to the study of personality than Meyer and Henderson. He rejected the psychoanalytic approach to personality, which he viewed as interpreting beyond the data, but was equally rejecting of the behavioural approach, which he considered did not interpret enough. In their place he developed a trait theory of personality. Before his theory was described, the word 'trait' was very liberally used to cover different types of behaviour, belief systems and habits, and was generally reviled as a scientific concept.

Allport (1927), together with his brother, Henry, the originator of social psychology (Allport and Allport, 1921), made trait theory respectable by defining it more tightly with five key elements:

(1) the recognition of 'trait' as the unit of personality,

(2) the admission of a probable hierarchy of traits, certainly of unit tendencies higher than the level of specific habits,

(3) an approach to the problem of the limits of generalization in the most comprehensive traits,

(4) the admission of both a major synthesis in personality as well as minor syntheses and dissociated acts,

(5) the tentative admission of subjective values as the core of such syntheses, but the exclusion of objective evaluation (character judgments) from purely psychological method.

(Allport, 1927)

The first two of these are the most significant. Traits were persistent; other features (unless they were linked to traits) were not, and so it was reasonable to regard the measurement of traits as a true record of personality. The second acknowledged that all trait measures were only a guide to underlying personality and that although relatively few 'higher order' traits might be identified, there were many other 'lower order' ones that could be measured too (covered by points 3 and 4 above). The fifth point allowed for the subjective expression of relevant traits to be more dominant than objective measures alone (e.g. the fact that you hit somebody after an argument did not necessarily mean you had an aggressive trait).

A single sentence tried to cover all these points:

A trait is a dynamic trend of behavior which results from the integration of numerous specific habits of adjustment, and which expresses a characteristic mode of the individual's reaction to his surroundings.

(Allport, 1927, p. 288).

But of course this chapter would be remiss if it pretended that the range of personality can be completely encapsulated by a single description or a set of traits. The best personality descriptions come from books, both fictional and biographical. Here is an excellent dissection of the differences in the writings of Charles Dickens and Leo Tolstoy that illustrates the subtleties of personality description:

Except in a rather roundabout way, one cannot learn very much from Dickens. And to say this is to think almost immediately of the great Russian novelists of the nineteenth century. Why is it that Tolstoy's grasp seems to be so much larger than Dickens's – why is it that he seems able to tell you so much more about yourself? It is not that he is more gifted, or even, in the last analysis, more intelligent. It is because he is writing about people who are growing. His characters are struggling to make their souls, whereas Dickens's are already finished and perfect. In my own mind Dickens's people are present far more often and far more vividly than Tolstoy's, but always in a single unchangeable attitude, like pictures or pieces of furniture. You cannot hold an imaginary conversation with a Dickens character as you can with, say, Peter Bezoukhov. [Note that Orwell hated using foreign words, so Pierre became Peter.]

(Orwell, 1940)

This is where descriptions of personality types can never do their subjects justice, and even traits go only part of the way to understanding. We need to assess personality abnormality, even within the bounds of a limited classification system, in a way that allows for considerable variation, rather than a stock display of characters that only appear to be cartoons. This shows the attraction of Dickens as a character builder but not as a developer. We need a classification of personality and personality disorder that allows people to grow or even shrink, like Tolstoy's, a daunting challenge.

1.3 Age 3. The Age of Investigation and Intervention

By the middle of the twentieth century there was a reasonable level of agreement between psychologists, psychiatrists and the lay public about personality. 'Habit is the fly-wheel of society', said William James (1890), and a tighter definition of 'habits' in the form of traits, and a general understanding that personality was a measurable entity helped research and discourse.

But since the time of Koch, paradoxically, the more personality disorder was studied, the more it was rejected. The main reason was that stigma had added its own carriage on the train of personality disorder and has been there ever since, waving furiously at bystanders to stay away. Pierre Janet added a little more by his description of the hysterical personality in 1893, essentially a fuller development of his idea of hysteria as dissociation. Kraepelin also described psycho-pathic personalities but was eclipsed by Kurt Schneider, who in 1923 attempted to synthesise previous descriptions in his book, *Die Psychopathischen Persönlichkeiten* (Schneider, 1923).

This described ten different personalities, not formally called disorders but certainly interpreted as such. It is often believed that he garnered his ideas from his clinical experience but he had already published a book on *The Personality and Fate of Registered Prostitutes* in 1921 (Schneider, 1921) when he described 12 different personality types. These types were all called 'psychopathic' and they have dominated the nomenclature for a century with no good justification (see Table 1.1). They had the asset of not being value laden and so were not prejudiced like Koch, but whether a classification based on clinical impressions alone, especially if they were primarily obtained in brothels in Hamburg, should dominate the field for a century is hard to understand. It is sometimes said that the eminence of a scientist can be measured by the number of years he or she holds up progress. On this basis Schneider is a gold medallist. If he had produced his classification of prostitutes today, the reception of his ideas would have been very different; he would have been macerated on Twitter.

Either because of Schneider, or simply because he wrote his book when the tide was at the flood, personality disorder research has steadily deviated from general personality research in the past century. Psychologists in the main, but many others too, have continued to study personality in accordance with trait theory as well as other models, and the development of the so-called Big Five (Table 1.2) is an example of this.

Psychiatrists in clinical practice have gone in a different direction down the Schneiderian path. Rather than carry out research to test the value and utility of this clinical/prostitution-derived classification, it has embraced it uncritically, changed a few names here and there, described each category as though it was unique and definitive when in fact it is swamped by comorbidity of other personality disorders, and then wonder why mixed personality disorder or PD-NOS (personality disorder – not otherwise specified) is so commonly used in practice (Verheul and Widiger, 2004). They have also introduced a gremlin into the system called borderline personality disorder. Here we cannot really blame Schneider alone, despite his adjective 'emotionally unstable' being attached to the condition. The circuitous route by which this was introduced to the classification is discussed in Chapter 4.

The influence of the psychoanalysts was considerable in denying empirical research into the personality disorder concept. Whereas Meyer had managed to straddle psychoanalysis

Table 1.1 The influence of Galen and Kurt Schneider on current classifications of personality disorder

Galen[a]	Schneider	DSM-IV-TR	ICD-6	ICD-10
Choleric	Emotionally unstable	Borderline	Emotional instability	Emotionally unstable, including borderline and impulsive
Choleric	Explosive	Antisocial	Antisocial	Dissocial
Choleric	Self-seeking	Narcissistic	...	...
Choleric	...	Histrionic	Immature	Histrionic
Melancholic	Depressive	Depressive[b]	Cyclothymic[cb]	...
Melancholic	Asthenic	Avoidant	Passive dependency	Anxious (avoidant)
Melancholic	Weak-willed	Dependent	Inadequate	Dependent
Phlegmatic	Affectless	Schizoid	Schizoid	Schizoid
Phlegmatic	...	Schizotypal	Asocial	...
Not classified elsewhere	Insecure sensitive	Paranoid	Paranoid	Paranoid
Not classified elsewhere	Insecure anankastic	Obsessive–compulsive	Anankastic	Anankastic
Not classified elsewhere	Fanatical	...	...	...
Sanguine	Hyperthymic	...	...	...

DSM=Diagnostic and Statistical Manual of Mental Disorders. ICD=International Classification of Diseases. [a] Galen produced *De Temperamentis* in AD 192; *De Temperamentis*. Edited and translated by P. N. Singer, P. J van der Eijk & P. Tassinari, 2019. Cambridge: Cambridge University Press. [b] A diagnosis listed in earlier versions of DSM and recommended for further study in DSM-IV. [c] This category appeared in later revisions of ICD and DSM but was subsequently recoded under affective (mood) disorders.

and biological psychiatry with some success, he still aimed for a scientific psychiatry that found out the causes, diagnosis and treatment of all mental illnesses. But after he died, the psychoanalysts, coming from a completely different tradition, abhorred the notion of any form of diagnostic labelling. In the end, in order to get their agreement to support DSM-III, Bob Spitzer, as we describe later, had, in effect, to buy them off by giving them personality disorder to do with as they pleased. This was realpolitik – it had nothing to do with science.

So personality disorder did not enter the mainstream of day-to-day psychiatric practice and classification principles have not caught up. What happens now is that only the most severe disorders are diagnosed, assessment becomes highly specialised, treatment becomes focused more on exclusion than inclusion, and the many people who at first feel heartened by the recognition of their problems are disillusioned by the limited interventions offered.

Table 1.2 Neuroticism, extraversion, agreeableness, conscientiousness, and openness
The Big Five (higher order) personality traits.

Personality feature	Essential elements at each extreme
Neuroticism	Calm and confident versus anxious, pessimistic and fearful
Extraversion	Sociable and fun-loving versus reserved and thoughtful
Agreeableness	Trusting, helpful and affable versus suspicious, uncooperative and hostile
Conscientiousness	Disciplined and careful versus impulsive and disorganised
Openness to experience	Likes routine, practical and predictable events versus imaginative and spontaneous ones

Although the epidemiologists have shown the size of the problems created by personality disorder (see Chapter 5), the subject remains seriously neglected. This particularly applies to research. Only a tiny proportion of funded research is allocated to personality disorder, the vast majority of it to the borderline condition. The antisocial group, despite incurring massive costs, remains stuck in a risk assessment time warp. It is sad to read the words of a distinguished author in the area: 'because there are no standard treatments of antisocial personality, it is essential to identify coexisting problems that *can* respond' (Black, 2013, p. 169). How many randomised trials have been mounted to investigate the value of new treatments in this condition? Read Chapter 8 to find out, and prepare to be shocked.

1.4 Age 4. The Age of Acceptance and Understanding

We hope this age is just about to start. Our hope is that the new ways of looking at personality disorder, especially the new ICD-11 classification and a broader awareness of the ubiquity of personality dysfunction, offer a way of bringing personality disorder back into the mainstream, as Adolf Meyer would have wanted. The recent history of personality disorder, if it tells us anything of value, informs us that the current road travelled has a dead end. We have to change course and come back together with our psychological colleagues. We need to make personality disorder respectable by emphasising we are all on the same spectrum of disturbance, embrace good trait theory, abolish useless categories that only confuse and mislead, and tread forward with a secure footing on the route outlined in this book. So we expect that all clinicians of the future will ask themselves the question, 'what about the personality', whenever they are assessing and planning the care of the patients they meet in their working lives.

Assessment of Personality
From Normal to Disorder

The two main reasons, we suspect, why most health professionals shy away from assessing personality status is that it is considered both too complicated and too risky. The risky aspect is discussed in Chapter 9 in dealing with stigma. In this chapter, the process of assessment is taken in stages in a form that everybody can appreciate without prior knowledge of the subject. Throughout the book we will be putting the main focus on the new ICD-11 classification of personality disorder, but the general principles of assessment apply to all ways of looking at personality disorder.

We are also assuming in this chapter that the reader has a fair knowledge of psychiatric assessment, but the first stages apply to all health professionals, including general practitioners, who are involved in patient care. The main message here is to emphasise that personality assessment is not just a task for the specialist.

2.1 Preliminary Stage

Six elements are essential when assessing personality (Table 2.1).

These six areas are covered in any good clinical assessment, and once the ancillary questions are answered the assessor should be able to at least make a rough impression of personality status. Please note that this assessment can be completed in a 20–30-minute clinical interview.

From this interview, it is relatively easy to place the person's current personality status on the scale above. Some will baulk at the idea that after a short interview it is possible to make an assessment of personality status, still less to disclose this to the patient. To use a comment on the MIND website: 'being given a diagnosis or label of personality disorder can feel as if you're being told there's something wrong with who you are' (MIND, 2020). The important two words here are 'can feel'. If the information is conveyed in the right way, it can be construed as valuable and positive.

The first task is to use the personality spectrum in Figure 2.1 to place the person at an approximate point. It will be extremely rare for anyone with severe personality disorder to be seen without clear evidence of serious dysfunction already being known, so the clinician is likely to be looking at placing the person somewhere on one of the three lower levels of severity, or in the no personality dysfunction group. One difficulty here will be in separating the problems created by current mental state symptoms from the difficulties of personality function. This is best clarified by checking on timescales. If the problems posed by personality difficulties are long-lasting (which they usually will be) and the mental state ones have clear beginnings and ends, then it is possible to conclude that the personality problems are likely to be independent. But in some instances (e.g. in chronic anxiety disorders beginning

Table 2.1 Essential first elements of personality assessment

Questions to ask after clinical assessment	Strands of relevant evidence	Follow-up questions
Is there any evidence of interpersonal social dysfunction?	Difficulties expressed in family/child/occupation during interview	Is this problem only with this person? Does it apply to others too?
Is the dysfunction persistent?	History of problem will indicate if same problem is repeated	How long (or how many times) has this problem lasted?
Does it only show itself in certain situations?	Determine places and times of difficulties	Would other people (in different situations) be aware of this?
Has the person the ability to perform appropriate societal roles?	Determine if present role is consistent with past training and education	Do you think you are working at the right level for you?
Is there any risk of harm to self or others?	History should include any episodes of violence or self-harm	What were the circumstances of these episodes? How often are/were they?
Are there other mental state problems?	If personality problems are conspicuous, there will almost certainly be evidence of other mental illness (and often this is how the person will present)	Do you think your difficulties with other people are linked to your other symptoms (of the relevant mental illness)?

	Personality difficulty	Mild personality disorder	Moderate personality disorder	Severe personality disorder
No evidence of dysfunction	Dysfunction in discrete settings	Persistent dysfunction but integrated life present	More severe problems with risk to self/others	Very severe breakdown of function

Figure 2.1 The full spectrum of personality. Note that all are on this spectrum somewhere.

in childhood), it may be more difficult. In these instances, it is easy to forget about the personality and decide on an anxiety diagnosis. For many reasons, including the unsatisfactory nature of the diagnosis of generalised anxiety disorder (Tyrer and Baldwin, 2006; Tyrer, 2018) as well as its treatment implications (see Chapter 10), it might be preferable to think of the personality diagnosis first.

It would be arrogant and wrong to recommend here exactly what should be said to the patient after this initial personality assessment has been made. Many would feel it wise to say nothing and just make an entry in the notes, but we have found that the following approach can be very effective:

> My assessment suggests you have (the current mental state problem) and this may be complicated by your personality (structure). I get the impression, but please correct me if I have it wrong, that you have long/always been a person with difficulties in relationships with (give examples), and this has not helped. Have I described this correctly?

These introductory remarks set off a dialogue that can correct or reinforce the initial impression. Very rarely, there is the angry question: 'Are you saying I have a personality disorder?' The best way of responding to this is to point out that all of us have personalities, and to varying degrees they can cause difficulties, so there is nothing particularly special about this line of questioning. At the end of the interview, assuming that you have concluded that there is some degree of personality disorder present, you can disclose this to the patient, not in terms of personality disorder but personality function. The only element of personality that can be assessed accurately at just one point in time is personality function, not disorder. This is a critical point, emphasised in more detail elsewhere (Tyrer et al., 2007), and it illustrates the great variation in personality status over time that is mentioned in Chapter 8. There is also good evidence that the more severe personality disorders (using ICD-11 notation) are more persistent than less severe ones over a 12-year period (Tyrer et al., 2016b), so a diagnosis lower in the spectrum should be regarded as more provisional than for severe disorders.

The way this should be communicated to the patient is along the lines of, 'At present your personality function is poor, in that it is contributing to your distress. We must take this into account in deciding how to help you.' You could also add, 'This does not mean that you necessarily have a personality disorder as this could easily change.'

Some people might well ask whether it is worthwhile going to all this trouble on the basis of inadequate information. The critical point here is that you are flagging up personality status at the initial interview and may need to return to this later. More importantly, it may influence choice of treatment (see Chapter 8). In the ICD-11 and DSM-5 classifications there is no Axis II, which used to be a separate axis for personality, and so there is a real danger that personality problems might be neglected altogether (Newton-Howes et al., 2015b). What unfortunately happens, far too often in practice, is that initial personality status is ignored and it is only when the patient has failed to respond as expected to treatment that a retrospective diagnosis is made of personality disorder. This is a slur on the diagnosis and is one of the main contributors to stigma.

In this chapter, we will be concentrating on assessments linked to the new classifications for personality disorder, ICD-11 and the alternative model for DSM-5. The original DSM-5 model was rejected by the American Psychiatric Association and placed in the category for further study; it has been only modified slightly and has been reinforced by additional empirical data. The DSM Alternative Model for Personality Disorder (AMPD) and ICD-11 classifications appear at first sight to be very different but in fact share many similarities.

2.2 Previous Classifications

At the time of writing the ICD-10 classification of personality disorder is still extant but will be replaced by ICD-11 on 1st January 2022. The radical change between the ICD-10 and

ICD-11 is the abolition of categorical diagnosis of personality disorder and its replacement by a single spectrum of personality pathology. The need for change was driven by the absence of empirical support for the 9–10 different categories, a massive degree of overlap between the criteria for different categories (wrongly described as comorbidity), the failure to use these categories in practice apart from borderline and emotionally unstable, with lesser support for antisocial and dissocial, and the wide use of 'mixed personality disorder' and 'personality disorder – not otherwise specified (personality disorder–NOS)' by clinicians who were just bemused by the confusing advice on offer.

All the existing categories of personality disorder will cease to exist in ICD after January 2022 with the exception of a 'borderline pattern specifier'. This, we stress again, is not a diagnosis but can be used by those who wish to maintain continuity with the old classification.

2.3 Diagnosis of Personality Disorder in ICD-11

2.3.1 Assessment of Severity

This is outlined above in principle but needs to be defined more clearly to determine the exact level of severity on the personality spectrum. Ideally every patient seen in clinical practice should be expected to have at least some assessment of personality status at an early stage. This would not just apply to psychiatrists but to all health professionals. In the present climate of stigma the implementation of this suggestion is a long way off, but it is still desirable. The reasons for making this suggestion are clarified in Chapters 7 and 8, as awareness of personality status should influence the treatment and management strategy being offered.

The severity spectrum is simple, and because it is so important it is presented here again (Figure 2.2).

The details of the classification are shown in Table 2.2. The most important difference distinguishing ICD-11 from ICD-10 is the complete absence of overlap with other personality groupings. Everybody, at any point in time, is in one place on Figure 2.2; it is impossible to be in more than one.

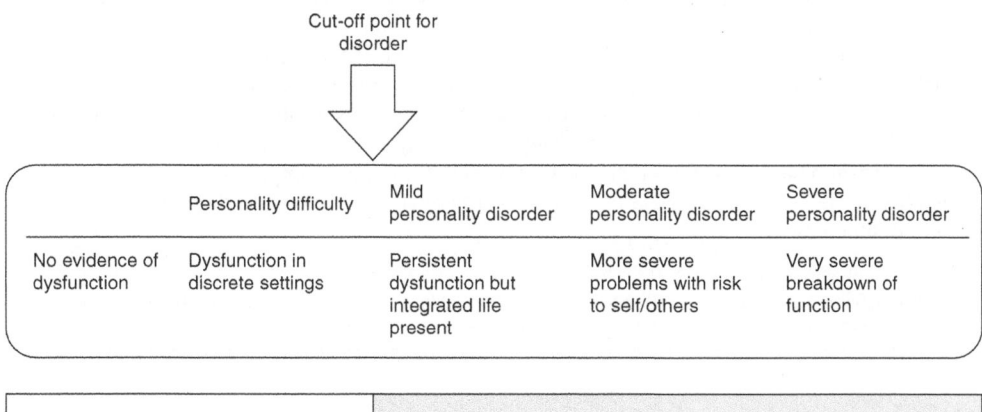

Figure 2.2 The need for a dichotomous separation of personality disorder for epidemiological purposes.

Table 2.2 The ICD-11 definitions for each level of severity of personality disorder.

Mild Personality Disorder

All general diagnostic requirements for Personality Disorder are met. Disturbances affect some areas of personality functioning but not others (e.g., problems with self-direction in the absence of problems with stability and coherence of identity or self-worth), and may not be apparent in some contexts. There are problems in many interpersonal relationships and/or in performance of expected occupational and social roles, but some relationships are maintained and/or some roles carried out. Specific manifestations of personality disturbances are generally of mild severity. Mild Personality Disorder is typically not associated with substantial harm to self or others, but may be associated with substantial distress or with impairment in personal, family, social, educational, occupational or other important areas of functioning that is either limited to circumscribed areas (e.g., romantic relationships; employment) or present in more areas but milder.

Moderate Personality Disorder

All general diagnostic requirements for Personality Disorder are met. Disturbances affect multiple areas of personality functioning (e.g., identity or sense of self, ability to form intimate relationships, ability to control impulses and modulate behaviour). However, some areas of personality functioning may be relatively less affected. There are marked problems in most interpersonal relationships and the performance of most expected social and occupational roles are compromised to some degree. Relationships are likely to be characterised by conflict, avoidance, withdrawal, or extreme dependency (e.g., few friendships maintained, persistent conflict in work relationships and consequent occupational problems, romantic relationships characterised by serious disruption or inappropriate submissiveness). Specific manifestations of personality disturbance are generally of moderate severity. Moderate Personality Disorder is sometimes associated with harm to self or others, and is associated with marked impairment in personal, family, social, educational, occupational or other important areas of functioning, although functioning in circumscribed areas may be maintained.

Severe Personality Disorder

All general diagnostic requirements for Personality Disorder are met. There are severe disturbances in functioning of the self (e.g., sense of self may be so unstable that individuals report not having a sense of who they are or so rigid that they refuse to participate in any but an extremely narrow range of situations; self-view may be characterised by self-contempt or be grandiose or highly eccentric). Problems in interpersonal functioning seriously affect virtually all relationships and the ability and willingness to perform expected social and occupational roles is absent or severely compromised. Specific manifestations of personality disturbance are severe and affect most, if not all, areas of personality functioning. Severe Personality Disorder is often associated with harm to self or others, and is associated with severe impairment in all or nearly all areas of life, including personal, family, social, educational, occupational, and other important areas of functioning.

(World Health Organization, 2018, 6D10 Personality disorder)
NB. The definition of personality difficulty is part of this classification and is described in Chapter 3. It is not included here as it is not a diagnosed psychiatric disorder.

2.3.2 Generic Definition of Personality Disorder

Although the ICD-11 classification is a radical change from ICD-10, the general description of personality disorder is remarkably similar in both classifications:

> Personality disorder is characterised by problems in functioning of aspects of the self (e.g., identity, self-worth, accuracy of self-view, self-direction), and/or interpersonal dysfunction (e.g., ability to develop and maintain close and mutually satisfying relationships, ability to understand others' perspectives and to manage conflict in relationships) that have persisted over an extended period of time (e.g., 2 years or more). The disturbance is manifest in patterns of cognition, emotional experience, emotional expression, and behaviour that are maladaptive (e.g., inflexible or poorly regulated) and is manifest across a range of personal and social situations (i.e., is not limited to specific relationships or social roles). The patterns of behaviour characterizing the disturbance are not developmentally appropriate and cannot be explained primarily by social or cultural factors, including socio-political conflict. The disturbance is associated with substantial distress or significant impairment in personal, family, social, educational, occupational or other important areas of functioning.
> (World Health Organization, 2018, 6D10 Personality disorder)

The most noteworthy difference is the phrase 'persisted over an extended period of time (e.g. 2 years or more)'. No timescale of onset is indicated, so in practice it is possible to diagnose personality disorder at any age from 10 to 100. The implications of this are discussed in Chapter 10.

All patients with mild, moderate and severe personality disorder have to satisfy the general description of the condition. The separation of the three further groups is shown in Table 2.2.

2.3.3 ICD-11 Trait Domain Qualifiers

The general view of those psychiatrists with a special interest in personality disorders, at least before 2010, was that the individual categories such as narcissistic, antisocial and borderline had clinical meaning and could not be linked to normal variation. This was expressed by the criticism of the ICD-11 proposal as promoting the 'still unproved idea that normal personality offers a valid bridge to the structure of abnormal personality' (Gunderson and Zanarini, 2011). At the same time, a large majority of general psychiatrists was expressing its views in a different way – by hardly ever diagnosing personality disorder.

The critical decision of the ICD-11 working group was to incorporate all personality disturbance into a single spectrum and to accept that the categories given credence by long standing had no intrinsic validity and should be abandoned. But in other ways some aspects of the categories were relevant and could be represented as domain traits. These could be then be used to qualify the level of severity of personality disorder.

This was difficult to accept for many. Although there was strong consensus that DSM-IV and ICD-10 personality disorder categories were unsatisfactory and should be replaced (Bernstein et al., 2007b), there was no consistency on what should be brought in to replace them (Mulder et al., 2011). Instead, there was a wide range of strongly held, often opposing, views. Some who commented, including a voluble group of patients, felt that all diagnoses of personality were stigmatising and should be discarded. There is partial justification for their views, as is explained in Chapters 9 and 10, but it is not a constructive option, except for some at low levels of personality disturbance who feel that their difficulties can be expressed differently. Others, including patients, researchers and clinicians, supported the existence of specific personality disorders, particularly the borderline category, and they were very concerned that it should remain in some form in any new classification (Bateman, 2011). Even those who advocated for one of the most overused phrases in science, a 'paradigm shift', had very different views on exactly what form this shift should take. This chapter reviews these positions and attempts to show that the ICD-11 system is the most relevant and accurate in its descriptions of personality pathology.

First, it is important to realise that early on, a conscious decision was made to separate the two issues of 'disorder' and 'behavioural manifestations'. The first part of this chapter discusses using severity as the marker of disorder. This part describes the behavioural manifestations. These replace the rigid categories in previous systems, none of which had any nosological status; all were clinical groupings decided by expert committees operating by opinion, not knowledge.

Second, the description of behavioural disturbance was constrained by the need for the descriptions to be reasonably concise, for practical reasons, as well as being clinically useful. The descriptors needed to be useful in all medical settings in all WHO countries and not just appeal to the small number of specialist personality disorder services. The importance of this cannot be overstated. Most descriptions of personality pathology were designed and used by personality disorder specialists who have the time and motivation to undertake comprehensive assessments, usually in high-income countries. In contrast, most working clinicians across the world do not have the luxury of time. We believe that an evidence-based simple classification is more likely to be used by a range of clinicians. Because, as we hope this book will show you, personality disorders are such important factors in treatment and outcome in mental and physical disorders, widespread use of basic personality descriptions is preferable to detailed assessments confined to specialists' clinics. In any case, specialist personality disorder clinics can always go beyond the ICD-11 categories if they wish.

Third, it was felt that linking personality disorder descriptors with models describing personality in community samples would be useful if evidence supported this. There is little doubt that personality pathology occurs on a continuum, however it is described. The logical consequence of this is that a dimensional descriptor of personality pathology would relate, in some way, to normally distributed personality dimensions.

Since the descriptors needed to be evidence-based, we systematically reviewed all studies which had explored the factor structure of patients with personality pathology. Our first observation was that the studies were very heterogeneous. They used different types of samples, including inpatients, outpatients and 'normal' subjects. They employed different models of personality pathology, varying methods to assess personality (including self-report and interviews) and subjected the findings to different statistical manipulations. Our second observation was that despite all their variability, the results were surprisingly consistent (Mulder et al., 2011).

All studies supported a general 'personality distress' dimension sharing common features such as generalised distress, low agreeableness, reduced flexibility and interpersonal difficulties. All studies also reported, in one form or another, two further dimensions. The first, usually largest with regard to explaining variance, is an externalising factor which incorporates symptoms then conceptualised as histrionic, narcissistic, borderline, anti-social and often paranoid personality disorder, in the ICD-10 and DSM-5 diagnostic systems.

The second factor, often called an internalising factor, is best represented as a mixture of avoidant and dependent personality disorder traits. Characteristics include shyness, anxious behaviour, pessimism and passivity.

Although not found in all studies, the third higher-order factor is what was generally conceptualised as schizoid behaviours: social indifference, aloofness and restricted expression of affect. In some studies, these behaviours overlapped with odd behaviours represented by schizotypal symptoms, in others, less so. Many people with this feature, as you might imagine, do not get included often in clinical studies.

A fourth factor also found in most, but not all, studies, was represented by obsessive-compulsive or anankastic symptoms and traits. In most studies which reported it, this factor was separated from the internalising factor. However, the factor seemed robust and relatively independent of all other symptoms of personality disorder.

Although these four factors were reported reasonably consistently across the reviewed studies and had good face validity, two problems were soon apparent. The first was that the externalising factor was broad and included important clinical symptoms conceptualised within the diagnoses of antisocial personality disorder and psychopathy. Traits such as callousness, lack of remorse and antisocial behaviour were part of externalising behaviours, but, some of the studies reported, loaded as a separate dimension (Dowson and Berrios, 1991; O'Boyle, 1995). After considerable debate within the ICD-11 group, a fifth factor, disinhibition, essentially trying to capture non-psychopathic externalising behaviours, was introduced for further study. This left the elephant in the room, borderline personality disorder, which despite being the most studied and venerated personality disorder, did not fit comfortably within any of these factors.

The ICD-11 proposal therefore consisted of five broad descriptions of personality pathology called trait domain qualifiers. These are not categorical syndromes but descriptive domains used 'to describe the characteristics of the individual that are most prominent and that contribute to personality disturbance' (World Health Organization, 2018, 6D11 Prominent personality traits or patterns). These domains, with some minor modifications, were accepted in ICD-11. They are described in Table 2.3 (https://icd.who.int/en).

2.4 Psychopathy and Personality Disorder

The word 'psychopath' has been used indiscriminately over the last 200 years in connection with personality disorder, but in recent years it has been focused on part of what is now the dissocial domain in ICD-11. The key authority in this area is Robert Hare, whose core publication, the Psychopathy Check List (revised version PCL-R, published in 2003), developed this in the 1970s after studying the pioneer work of Hervey Cleckley (1941). Cleckley identified 21 characteristics of psychopathy entirely from his clinical experience. Many of these became part of Hare's Psychopathy Check List, particularly in its revision in 2003 (PCL-R):

Cleckley's original 21 items comprising the essentials of psychopathy (Cleckley, 1941)

1 Superficial attractiveness (glibness/superficial charm[a])
2 Apparently free from any neurotic or psychotic symptom
3 Little or no sense of personal responsibility (irresponsibility[a])
4 Disregard for the truth (pathological lying[a])
5 Does not accept blame for their actions (failure to accept responsibility for own actions[a])
6 Has no sense of shame (lack of remorse or guilt[a])

Table 2.3 ICD-11 Prominent personality traits or patterns

6D11.0 Negative affectivity in personality disorder or personality difficulty

The core feature of the Negative Affectivity trait domain is the tendency to experience a broad range of negative emotions. Common manifestations of Negative Affectivity, not all of which may be present in a given individual at a given time, include: experiencing a broad range of negative emotions with a frequency and intensity out of proportion to the situation; emotional lability and poor emotion regulation; negativistic attitudes; low self-esteem and self-confidence; and mistrustfulness.

6D11.1 Detachment in personality disorder or personality difficulty

The core feature of the Detachment trait domain is the tendency to maintain interpersonal distance (social detachment) and emotional distance (emotional detachment). Common manifestations of Detachment, not all of which may be present in a given individual at a given time, include: social detachment (avoidance of social interactions, lack of friendships, and avoidance of intimacy); and emotional detachment (reserve, aloofness, and limited emotional expression and experience).

6D11.2 Dissociality in personality disorder or personality difficulty

The core feature of the Dissociality trait domain is disregard for the rights and feelings of others, encompassing both self-centeredness and lack of empathy. Common manifestations of Dissociality, not all of which may be present in a given individual at a given time, include: self-centeredness (e.g. sense of entitlement, expectation of others' admiration, positive or negative attention-seeking behaviours, concern with one's own needs, desires and comfort and not those of others); and lack of empathy (i.e., indifference to whether one's actions inconvenience hurt others, which may include being deceptive, manipulative, and exploitative of others, being mean and physically aggressive, callousness in response to others' suffering, and ruthlessness in obtaining one's goals).

6D11.3 Disinhibition in personality disorder or personality difficulty

The core feature of the Disinhibition trait domain is the tendency to act rashly based on immediate external or internal stimuli (i.e., sensations, emotions, thoughts), without consideration of potential negative consequences. Common manifestations of Disinhibition, not all of which may be present in a given individual at a given time, include: impulsivity; distractibility; irresponsibility; recklessness; and lack of planning.

6D11.4 Anankastia in personality disorder or personality difficulty

The core feature of the Anankastia trait domain is a narrow focus on one's rigid standard of perfection and of right and wrong, and on controlling one's own and others' behaviour and controlling situations to ensure conformity to these standards. Common manifestations of Anankastia, not all of which may be present in a given individual at a given time, include: perfectionism (e.g., concern with social rules, obligations, and norms of right and wrong, scrupulous attention to detail, rigid, systematic, day-to-day routines, hyper-scheduling and planfulness, emphasis on organisation, orderliness, and neatness); and emotional and behavioural constraint (e.g., rigid control over emotional expression, stubbornness and inflexibility, risk-avoidance, perseveration, and deliberativeness).

(World Health Organization, 2018)

7 'Undependable' – cheats and lies without any compunction (pathological lying[a])

8 'Execrable' judgement

9 Inability to learn or profit from experience (lack of realistic long-term goals[a])

10 Gross egocentricity (grandiose sense of self-worth[a])

11 Poverty of affect with no depth of feeling (shallow affect[a])

12 Lacking insight cannot see self as others see them (callous/lacking empathy[a])

13 No appreciation for kindness or consideration shown by others (parasitic lifestyle[a])

14 Alcohol indulgences

15 When drinking 'places self in disgraceful or ignominious position seeking a state of stupefaction

16 Not suicidal

17 Sex life shows peculiarities with interest in casual sex (promiscuous sexual behaviour[a])

18 No evidence of familial inferiority or heredity

19 No evidence of early maladjustment

20 Inability to follow any plan consistently

21 Has a life plan that ends in failure

[a]Concepts that have been retained in Hare's PCL-R (2003) instrument.

Apart from the alcohol elements, not now considered to be unrelated to personality directly (but see Chapter 7), most of these items constitute the PCL-R.

The PCL-R has become the lodestone of psychopathy. A score on the scale of 30 is said to be diagnostic of psychopathy and one between 25 and 29 being strongly indicative of the disorder. How does this square with moderate and severe personality disorder in the ICD-11 classification?

The conclusion reached by our ICD-11 working group was that the case to have psychopathy introduced as a separate domain in the classification was very weak. The main features of classical Cleckleyan psychopathy were all encapsulated within the dissociality domain. This conclusion chimes with the conclusion of Essi Viding, who has performed ground-breaking work on the genetics of personality disturbance in childhood. There has been much interest in callous and unemotional traits in young people, and the Viding group have suggested that it is these traits that are genetically determined and might be the core of psychopathy (Viding et al., 2005). But despite this, Essi Viding (2019) has concluded that the domain of psychopathy, although having some elements particular to its own, lies within the area of antisociality. There are small differences – Venables et al. (2014) show the core psychopath has more 'boldness' – but much of this can be explained by native intelligence. A cunning and manipulative classical psychopath is much more likely to impress than a 20 year recidivist who is trying to con.

The finding of a genetic component to psychopathy is also important to notice, as ever since Lee Robins' influential book (1966) on the long-term outcome of childhood deviance there has been a tendency to overplay early environment as the main instigator of adult antisocial behaviour and the consequent term 'sociopathy'. As Viding puts it, 'the genetic propensity is of course not a destiny, but again highlights the fact that there are children who are more vulnerable than others and we should not shy away from identifying and helping them. I think "personality disorder in development" could be a helpful development in this regard' (E. Viding 2020, personal communication, 14 December 2020).

Table 2.4 ICD-11 Definition of borderline personality disorder

6D11.5 Borderline pattern

The Borderline pattern descriptor may be applied to individuals whose pattern of personality disturbance is characterised by a pervasive pattern of instability of interpersonal relationships, self-image, and affects, and marked impulsivity, as indicated by many of the following: Frantic efforts to avoid real or imagined abandonment; A pattern of unstable and intense interpersonal relationships; Identity disturbance, manifested in markedly and persistently unstable self-image or sense of self; A tendency to act rashly in states of high negative affect, leading to potentially self-damaging behaviours; Recurrent episodes of self-harm; Emotional instability due to marked reactivity of mood; Chronic feelings of emptiness; Inappropriate intense anger or difficulty controlling anger; Transient dissociative symptoms or psychotic-like features in situations of high affective arousal.

(World Health Organization, 2018)

2.5 What about Borderline Personality Disorder?

As noted previously, borderline personality disorder symptoms have a complex relationship with the ICD-11 model, and with all personality trait models. As discussed in Chapter 4, borderline personality disorder did not emerge from personality trait models and most features of borderline personality disorder are clinical symptoms rather than personality traits (Tyrer, 2009b). No factor analytic studies have supported a categorical borderline personality disorder factor (Sharp, 2016). It seems better to regard borderline personality disorder as a general personality factor (Sharp et al., 2015), possibly related to severity. Within the ICD-11 domains, it is strongly related to disinhibition and negative affectivity and moderately related to dissociality.

Nevertheless, despite this overwhelming evidence, challenging the existence of borderline personality disorder led to alarm. In particular, clinicians specialising in the treatment of borderline personality disorder, especially those with substantial research grants, supported strongly the retention of the diagnosis in its present form. They pointed out that borderline personality disorder was the most researched personality disorder category with regard to treatment and aetiology (Herpertz et al., 2017), and it should be retained regardless of its validity. A political compromise was eventually reached with the ICD-11 Classification Committee and an optional 'borderline pattern qualifier' was added to the five domains. This is defined in Table 2.4.

2.6 Measurement of ICD-11 Domains: Reliability and Validity

Because ICD-11 has only just been approved by the World Health Organization, instruments to measure severity and domains have only been developed very recently. Initial reliability and validity studies used older diagnostic measures. A Korean study using DSM-IV personality disorder symptoms reported that the anankastic, detached and dissocial domains were coherent and discriminated well. However, the other two domains, emotionally unstable and anxious/dependent (as they were then called), were less robust and seemed to be more diffuse (Kim et al., 2015). In a large sample of 606 depressed outpatients, DSM-IV personality disorder symptoms were independently assigned by two raters to the five ICD-11 domains and a confirmatory factor analysis in an exploratory framework was used.

The best fitting model produced five domains with anankastic, detached and dissocial domains closely matching the ICD-11 proposal. The negative affectivity and disinhibition domains were less distinctly represented (Mulder et al., 2016), but it should be mentioned that not many of the relevant terms for these items appear in the DSM classification.

Bo Bach and colleagues developed an ICD-11 trait domain algorithm for the Personality Inventory for DSM-5 (PID-5), a diagnostic instrument developed for the DSM-5 Alternative Model for Personality Disorders (AMPD) which has been widely used. They reported that the ICD-11 and AMPD domains were largely compatible. The ICD-11 traits were organised in a hierarchal structure with a single personality disorder pathology domain at the top and the five ICD-11 domains at the lower level (Figure 2.3) (Bach et al., 2017).

A further study in psychiatric outpatients showed relative continuity with traditional categorical personality disorders and captured most of their information (Bach et al., 2018). Further support for the initial structural validity of ICD-11 has come from an Iranian sample (Lotfi et al., 2018).

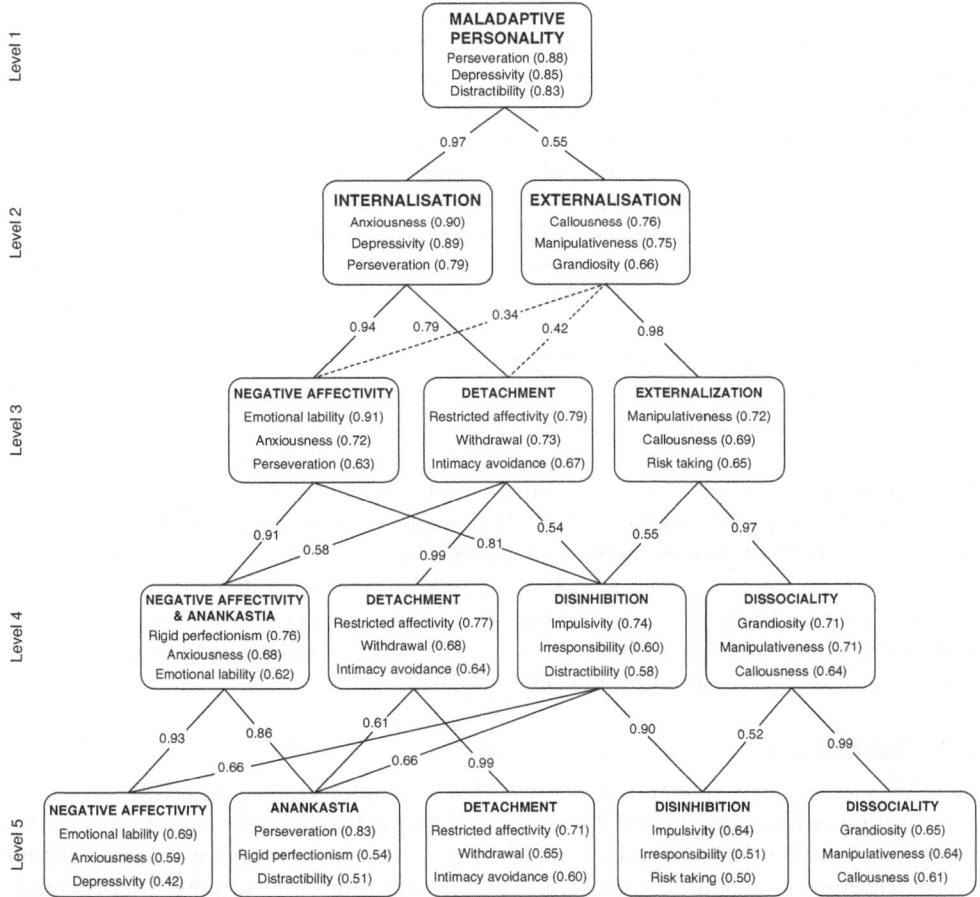

Figure 2.3 The hierarchical structure of personality disturbance. (Bach et al., 2017)

Bach and colleagues also used the PID-8 to allocate ICD-11 trait domains in a group of 226 patients who had been diagnosed using the 10 traditional personality disorder categories. The relationship between traditional DSM-5 personality disorders and ICD-11 domains is shown in Table 2.5 from their paper (Bach et al., 2018).

The relationships are largely as predicted. Of note is that borderline personality disorder and paranoid personality disorder are moderately to strongly correlated with all ICD-11 domains.

More recently, instruments which attempt to measure the ICD-11 personality disorder classification model have been developed. The Standardised Assessment of Severity of Personality Disorder (SASPD) (Olajide et al., 2018) was modelled after the Standardised Assessment of Personality – Abbreviated Scale (Moran et al., 2003). It has nine items which are linked to the five ICD-11 domains. Each item is measured on a four-point scale (see Chapter 10).

The Personality Inventory for ICD-11 (PiCD) is a 60-item self-report measuring the five trait domains. Each domain has 12 items rated from 1 (strongly disagree) to 5 (strongly agree). More recently, an Informant-Report Form of the PiCD (Bach et al., 2020a) and a modified PID5F which measures ICD-11 and DSM-5 trait domains (Bach et al., 2020b) have been developed.

Several studies have examined the psychometric properties of these scales. In general, they have reported that the domains exhibit adequate internal consistency (Gutiérrez et al., 2015; Carnovale et al., 2019). Factor analyses have supported the ICD-11 structure with the notable exception that some studies find four factors rather than five. The anankastia and disinhibition domains are organised along a bipolar dimension (Gutiérrez et al., 2015; Carnovale et al., 2019; Bach et al., 2020b). However, other studies support a five factor solution in which anankastia and disinhibition are two distinct domains (Mulder et al., 2016; Bach et al., 2017). The clinical reality may be that complex personality disorder patterns can be characterised by both disinhibition and anankastia (Chamberlain et al., 2018).

The other major point is that the PiCD domains moderately overlap. While some may see this as a disadvantage, it probably reflects the true nature of personality traits. The PiCD domains average correlations are similar to those of DSM-5 taxonomy and the Big Five personality traits (Saucier, 2002; Gutiérrez et al., 2019) and overlap between personality domains focus on integral part of a repeatedly replicated structure (Markon et al., 2005).

We initially proposed that the five ICD-11 domains might be aligned with the five-factor model (FFM) in the following manner: negative affectivity with neuroticism, detachment with low extraversion, dissocial with low agreeableness, disinhibited with low conscientiousness and anankastia with high conscientiousness (Mulder et al., 2016). In general, these relationships have been supported. Table 2.6 shows the correlations between the PiCD scales and FFM scales in a sample of over 1,000 Italian adults.

2.7 Summary

The ICD-11 classification of personality disorders is a radical change from ICD-10; it offers a wholly dimensional system and discards all existing categories. The exception is the late retention of the borderline specifier, which is not part of the evidence-based model but whose removal was seen as too large a loss by various groups of researchers in personality disorders as well as a proportion of clinicians. The utility of the borderline specifier within

Table 2.5 Bivariate associations of ICD-11 personality trait domains with personality disorder criterion count

| | SCID-II rated personality disorders | | | | | | | | | |
| | Cluster A | | | Cluster B | | | | Cluster C | | |
	PAR	SCD	STY	ANT	BOR	HIS	NAR	AVO	DPT	OBS
Negative affectivity	**0.45**	0.06	0.33	−0.09	**0.51**	**0.29**	0.05	**0.54**	**0.46**	**0.23**
Detachment	**0.43**	**0.46**	**0.41**	0.26	0.38	0.04	0.23	0.33	0.17	0.15
Dissociality	**0.52**	0.31	0.36	**0.60**	0.43	0.32	**0.71**	0.00	0.06	0.26
Disinhibition	0.47	0.28	0.44	**0.49**	**0.60**	**0.43**	0.45	0.18	0.34	0.13
Anankastia	0.44	0.22	0.40	0.15	0.48	0.34	0.25	0.35	0.24	**0.62**

Boldfaced correlations indicate the hypothesised trait domains for each personality disorder type.
(Bach et al., 2018)

Table 2.6 The *Personality Inventory for ICD-11 Scales: Correlations (i.e. Pearson r values) with the Five Factor Personality Model Index Scores* (N = 1,122).

Five Factor Model Personality Index subscales	M	SD	Stratified α	Personality inventory for ICD-11 scale r values				
				NA	DT	DL	DN	AN
Neuroticism	.00	.89	.85	<u>.81</u>	.30	.15	.38	-.03
Extraversion	.00	.91	.89	-.34	<u>-.73</u>	.04	-.09	-.12
Agreeableness	.00	.94	.90	-.15	-.37	<u>-.48</u>	-.20	.03
Conscientiousness	.00	.90	.83	-.28	-.22	-.08	<u>-.63</u>	<u>.44</u>
Openness to experience	.00	.94	.89	-.01	-.21	.07	.06	-.03

Note. ICD-11 = International Classification of Diseases, 11th Revision; NA = Negative Affective; DT = Detachment; DL = Dissocial; DN = Disinhibition; AN = Anankastic. For each Five Factor Index subscale, the stratified α coefficient was computed using sums of standardised scores of the Big Five Inventory and five factor model Rating Form corresponding scale. The expected convergent validity (i.e. Pearson r) coefficients between the Personality Inventory for ICD-11 scales and the Five-Factor Model Personality Index scales are underlined. The nominal significance level (i.e. $p < .05$) of Pearson r coefficients was corrected according to the Bonferroni procedure for multiple comparisons and set at $p < .002$. Pearson r values > |.09| are significant at $p < .002$. Bold highlights large effect size correlations ($r > |.50|$). (Somma et al., 2019) the domain structure remains unclear. Its early study does not appear promising (Mulder et al., 2020), but the subject is ripe for further investigation.

Despite criticism that the classification is too simple, the combination of a severity diagnosis and a mixture of any of the five domains offers many diagnostic options (over 200) and to date the general structure has been generally supported by researchers and clinicians. A number of questionnaires have been developed to measure the domains. They have generally supported the validity of the five-domain maladaptive trait model in ICD-11. The major question is that two of the domains (anankastia and disinhibition) may represent opposite poles of the same higher order domain. How to represent this within the model is the subject of some debate, not least as it is quite possible for all five domains to coexist in the same personality disordered patient.

The remaining chapters in this book will use the ICD-11 system wherever possible but will obviously have to refer to past research with the former classification structure. But whenever we can link past data and descriptions to ICD-11, we will do so. Despite some difference in terminology, it is not difficult for the practitioner to recognise the traditional categories of personality disorder in the following pages. Later chapters discuss the potential clinical utility of the model and describe clinicians' attitudes to the new structure; they have been positive to date.

We also want to widen the classification to all practitioners, irrespective of their status in medicine. There is the option of making a general diagnosis of personality disorder without necessarily adding trait domains. This does not suggest that the diagnosis can be attributed casually. It is just that when a practitioner feels that there is pathology beyond symptoms and interpersonal disturbance is prominent, the flag of personality disorder should be raised.

Although, as members of the ICD-11 revision group for personality disorders, we are clearly going to support its use, once it is being used in practice we are confident its value will be appreciated. But as we are always remembering evidence, more work is required before we can truly evaluate its validity and utility in clinical work.

Personality Difficulty

The term 'personality difficulty' will be unfamiliar to most people except as a general concept, but it will be part of the ICD-11 diagnostic spectrum of personality disorder in January 2022. We know a fair deal about it, but it is not a diagnosis. It is listed in the section of the ICD-11 classification for 'non-disease entities that constitute factors, influencing health status and encounters with health services, that may be of clinical importance', called Q Factors. The important section for personality difficulty is QE50 (problems associated with relationships). The full QE50 list is shown in Table 3.1.

Once personality difficulty has been recognised, it can be further qualified using codes for the same domain traits as personality disorders (Table 3.2). More than one of these can be selected if necessary.

Personality difficulty has some connections to the ICD-10 (Z-code) non-disorder category Z73.1 'accentuation of personality traits' which is a subcategory of the Z73 'Problems Related to Life-Management Difficulty' in the chapter 'Factors Influencing Health Status and Contact with Health Services' (World Health Organization, 1992). The reason why this is not a footnote to diagnosis but an important sub-syndromal diagnosis is that it is an integral part of the personality spectrum. It can create considerable disturbance in function and relationships, but it is generally easier to manage than personality disorder and its effects are not generalised.

3.1 Distinction between Personality Difficulty and Personality Disorder

Personality difficulty is similar to personality disorder in that it is characterised by relatively stable difficulties (e.g. at least 2 years) and can be recognised at any time of life. But there are important differences also (Table 3.3).

It is worth stressing again that personality difficulty is not a diagnosis and so cannot be denoted as such, but this does not mean it can be ignored. It can be a potent part of a diagnostic formulation.

This is because it (a) is remarkably common, (b) has an influence on the outcome of other mental disorders and (c) fluctuates over time and can change into a formal personality disorder (and vice versa) (Yang et al., 2021). People with personality difficulty also make greater use of health services and others in the population, have less good social function and are less likely to lead happy and contented lives (Tyrer, 2020b).

These conclusions have to be qualified as the data available have largely been extrapolated from existing studies. The evidence that personality difficulty is common comes from a large national study from the United Kingdom. The UK 2000 National Morbidity Survey

Table 3.1 Coding of personality difficulty in ICD-11

Q factor	Nature of problem
50.0	Problems associated with a relationship with a friend
50.1	Problems in relationships with teachers or classmates
50.2	Problems associated with relationships with people at work
50.3	Problems in relationships with neighbours, tenant or landlord
50.4	Problems in relationships with parents, in-laws or other family members
50.5	Problems related to discord with counsellors
50.6	Problems related to inadequate social skills
50.7	Personality difficulty

Table 3.2 Further coding of personality difficulty in ICD-11

Q factor	Nature of problem
6D11.0	Negative affectivity in personality disorder or personality difficulty
6D11.1	Detachment in personality disorder or personality
6D11.2	Dissociality in personality disorder or personality difficulty
6D11.3	Disinhibition in personality disorder or personality difficulty
6D 11.4	Anankastia in personality disorder or personality difficulty

Table 3.3 Differences between personality difficulty and disorder

Personality difficulty	Personality disorder
Intermittent presentation	Persistent presentation
Confined to certain situations	Present in all situations
Does not interfere greatly with normal social and occupational performance	Impairs social and occupational performance
Not associated with risk of harm to self or others	Often associated with risk of harm to self or others

assessed nearly 8,400 people, carefully chosen as representative of the population, using a statistical selection of postcodes. The respondents were assessed for both personality status and mental health. Personality assessment was made in a two-stage process using the Screening Version of the Structured Clinical Interview for DSM-IV (SCID) (Spitzer et al., 1990), and so represents a reasonably accurate record of personality status, even though it tends to overdiagnose personality disorder by about 20% (Ekselius et al., 1994). In the analysis, all people who had a score of one operational criterion less than the number needed to diagnose a SCID personality diagnosis received the personality difficulty label. So, for example, five criteria in the DSM definition of borderline personality disorder are needed to receive the diagnosis of borderline personality disorder, but a score of 4 would lead to the diagnosis of personality difficulty. The same process was applied to diagnose personality difficulty for each of the other personality disorders.

Reaching a sub-syndromal diagnosis of personality difficulty made in this way led to an astonishing figure; nearly half the respondents (48.3%) had this condition in the national survey (Yang et al., 2010). People with personality difficulty were more likely to consult their general practitioners, be admitted to mental hospital, attend a community mental health centre and see a social worker or community nurse, than others with no personality difficulty. This shows we are not dealing with a trivial condition that has no impact. Of course, if we allow for over-diagnosis by 20%, then the proportion would fall to 38%, but this is still a very large proportion of the adult population.

A similar study by a Finnish group (Karukivi et al., 2017), also using the SCID, this time in its complete version, with 352 patients, again using the cut-off point one below the official diagnosis, also showed very similar results. Patients with personality difficulty had more mental health problems and poorer functioning than those without personality difficulty.

In another study, the Nottingham Study of Neurotic Disorder, the long-term impact of personality difficulty on the outcome of anxiety and depression in a clinical population was assessed. This study was a randomised controlled trial, initially lasting for 10 weeks, and personality status, including personality difficulty, was evaluated using the Personality Assessment Schedule (Tyrer and Alexander, 1979; Tyrer et al., 1988). In the short term, personality status had no impact on outcome (Tyrer et al., 1990), but after the two-year assessment those diagnosed as personality difficulty at baseline had somewhat worse scores on the Comprehensive Psychopathological Rating Scale (a general measure of psychopathology) than those with no baseline personality dysfunction, and at 30 years had mean scores in the clinical diagnostic range (Figure 3.1). It is important to note that the personality problems in this group of patients were not addressed in treatment, only the symptomatic ones. Between 12% and 20% of all patients assessed as having personality difficulty at baseline also developed personality disorder at follow-up (Yang et al., 2021).

We cannot yet know if forthcoming studies would lead to the same results. At present the new instruments being developed for ICD-11 do not include personality difficulty. These include the Standardised Assessment of Severity of Personality Disorder (SASPD) (Olajide et al., 2018), the Personality Inventory for ICD-11 (PiCD) (Oltmanns and Widiger, 2019) and the Personality Assessment Questionnaire for ICD-11 (PAQ-11) (Kim et al., 2021). There is a new instrument in preparation, the Structured Clinical Interview for ICD-11 that is likely to include both personality disorder and difficulty in its coding.

But the opportunity of investigating the prevalence and impact of personality difficulty is easily available. For example, the SASPD has a cut-off point of 8 to diagnose mild personality disorder (Olajide et al., 2018), the least severe form of personality disorder. A score of 7 could be regarded as indicative of personality difficulty and data collected accordingly. But this needs further testing.

In Chapters 8 and 10 of this book, we give other instances where personality difficulty may be of clinical importance. We know from an initial study that the 'diagnosis' is easy to make in practice (Bach and First, 2018); what is needed now is further evidence of its value in the personality spectrum.

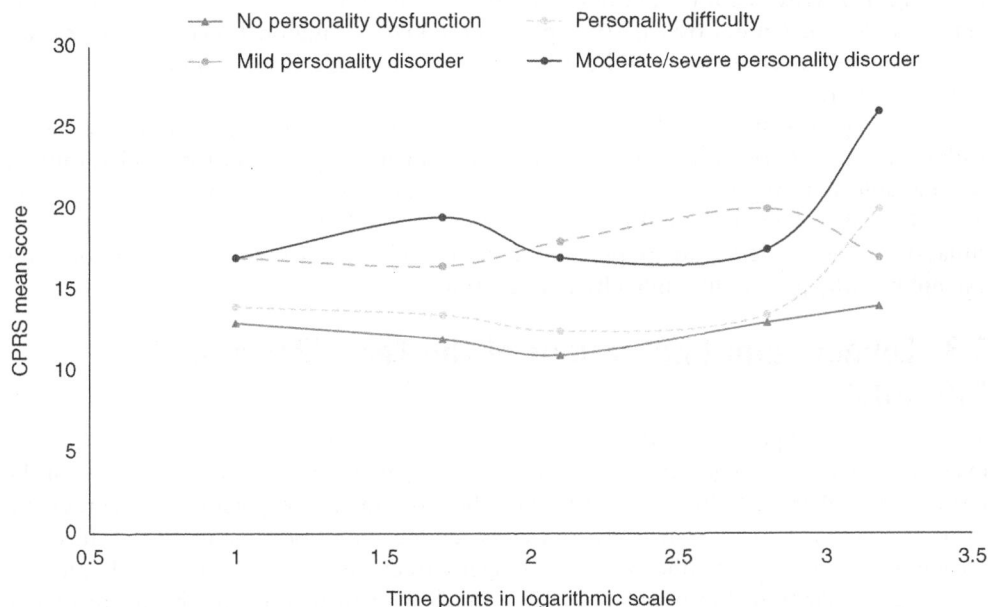

Figure 3.1 Long-term outcome of patients with personality difficulty who also had anxiety and depressive disorders. The period covers 30 years of follow-up and the x-axis is shown on a logarithmic scale to allow better interpretation of differences in the clinical data, which illustrate the mean scores on a global psychopathology scale (Comprehensive Psychopathological Rating Scale, CPRS). The follow-up times are 10 weeks, 1, 2, 12 and 30 years. Note that personality difficulty identified at baseline still has an influence on outcome at 30 years. (From Tyrer et al., in press. Figure reproduced by permission of the Editors of Psychological Medicine).

3.2 DSM and Levels of Personality Function

When the DSM-5 Alternative Model was being introduced, researchers recognised that severity of disorder had not been adequately addressed and the Level of Personality Functioning Scale (LPFS) was developed after further empirical analyses. This scale includes two primary areas of function, the self-domain, separated into identity and self-direction, and interpersonal functioning, separated into empathy and intimacy (Bender et al., 2011; Morey et al., 2011). As might be expected from their names, identity concerns autonomy and self-awareness, self-direction is linked to goal-setting and self-understanding, empathy encompasses the perspectives of others and one's own impact on them, and intimacy records both close relationships and the ability to relate well to others. Each scale is rated between 0 and 4 on the basis of impairment, with 0 at the least level of impairment. Although the Level of Personality Functioning Scale is only one part of the DSM-5 assessment, a rating of personality difficulty could readily be made from this scale. A shorter version, the Level of Personality Functioning Scale – Brief Form, of 20 items, has also been described and may be more useful in ordinary clinical practice (Weekers et al., 2019).

Overall, there are many ways in which personality difficulty can be recorded in ordinary practice and should always be thought of if any assessment falls short of a full personality disorder diagnosis. When critics cavil at a condition that allegedly affects a large proportion of the population on the grounds that it must represent over-diagnosis, we would just ask them to look at their own experiences. We all know colleagues who cause us to suffer. John

Eagles (2017) writes about a fictitious one in his fine novel about a junior psychiatrist, *Starting to Shrink*. (Junior psychiatrists, please note.) Dr Burlington, his consultant, is rude, patronising and overbearing, and humiliates his juniors with put-you-down faux psychoanalytical interpretations.

He may be very different elsewhere and is clearly successful in his career, but in dealing with his judged inferiors, he satisfies all the requirements of personality difficulty, causing considerable suffering to others (how many of his juniors have given up the profession because of his behaviour?), and persistently showing these features in these occupational situations. Most readers who are psychiatrists will have come across a Dr Burlington. This exemplifies why personality difficulty is so common.

3.3 Longer Term Implications of the Term 'Personality Difficulty'

The importance of personality difficulty will only become important in psychiatric thinking over time. Once all can get used to the concept of a personality spectrum the value of the term will be enhanced. When the swirls of doubt about the name 'personality disorder' are dispensed, and it is realised that most of us have a degree of personality disturbance, the attribution of personality difficulty will no longer attract any form of stigma as it is attached to a large minority of the population. How much it disturbs the equilibrium of society remains to be seen. We would also like to think that a little bit of personality difficulty makes us all more interesting people, and at some point we might even boast about it rather than hide it in a corner.

Borderline Personality Disorder
A Condition That Appeared Without Trace

Borderline Personality Disorder (BPD) is the most prominent and well recognised of all current personality disorder (PD) categories. However, it has not always been this way. In fact, the 'borderline patient' is one of the newer categories in personality classification. The term emerged, largely in North America, in the 1950s. While most 'psychopathic' personality types have been recognised in one form or another since the nineteenth century, borderline has not. Schneider's (see Chapter 1) classification, which formed much of the basis for the DSM-II and ICD-9 classification of personality, describes an 'emotionally unstable personality', but this is largely related to unstable mood and better translated as 'with labile mood' (*Stimmungslabile*). 'Explosive personality' shares some features with BPD, but these are confined to disinhibition. Kraepelin expanded pathological personalities to seven types in the eighth edition (1909–15) of his textbook, but only one – 'The Excitable' (*die Erregbaren*) – has any overlap with BPD.

The borderline personality, curiously, did not emerge from any pre-existing model of personality, even though the psychoanalysts claim it. The term was one of several used for describing patients lying on the border between neurosis and psychosis. It was chosen over other terms such as 'ambulatory schizophrenia', 'as-if' personality, 'pseudoneurotic schizophrenia' and 'borderline syndrome' (Perry and Klerman, 1978). Although the term 'borderline' had been used by authors such as Schmideberg in the 1940s, it referred to patients who were considered 'early cases of schizophrenia or near-schizophrenia' (Schmideberg, 1947, p. 45). The modern concept of the borderline patient emerged with Robert Knight's paper published in 1953 (Knight, 1953). He wrote that some neurotic or even near normal patients developed psychotic symptoms during psychoanalysis. He proposed criteria, focused on ego weakness, such as inappropriate affect, impaired concept formation, suspiciousness and obliviousness to the presence of these symptoms. He did not consider borderline as a PD but rather a clinical state related to schizophrenia which had a time-limited transient quality (Knight, 1953). Robert Knight was an influential figure, holding posts including president of the American Psychiatric Association and the American Psychoanalytic Association, and in some ways it is surprising that not more was made of this paper at the time.

There was no mention of a clear personality component in Knight's paper, but a shift occurred in the 1960s with an emphasis on the borderline patient being described as having enduring qualities more akin to a characterological flaw, or a personality disorder, by several writers. These included Otto Kernberg (Kernberg, 1967), who subsequently became the most influential. Building on Knight's ideas around impaired ego functioning, Kernberg constructed a complex model of personality organisation with the borderline patient postulated as functioning at an intermediate phase between neurosis and psychosis. His criteria included a shift towards primary process thinking, specific defences including splitting, projection and denial as well as pathological internalised object ideations. Kernberg went on to describe manifestations of ego weakness which are more consistent with current descriptors of BPD. These included poor anxiety tolerance leading to distress and possible acting out behaviour, a lack of impulse control and a deficit of sublimatory channels for patients' drives. Knight and Kernberg's models have very little in common and, in particular, the move from a mental state disorder to a personality disorder was not made with any conviction. Both descriptions were based on clinical observations and inferential judgement.

By contrast, Grinker and colleagues attempted to conduct research on a group of 51 patients considered borderline but not schizophrenic. They subjected the measures of ego functioning made in this group to a cluster analysis and identified four subtypes. These were (1) the psychotic border; (2) the core borderline syndrome; (3) the adaptive, affectless, defended, as-if persons; and (4) the border with neuroses. They noted that anger was the main affect with defects in affectional relationships and an absence of consistent self-identity (Grinker et al., 1968). Now, for the first time we had a clear notion of what the borderline concept was: a mixture of quasi-psychotic features, emotional instability, dissociative elements with outbursts of anger and the common symptoms of neurosis. Like a Russian doll, once you had evaluated one component, another appeared below, and still more at different times. So it was easy to see how the name 'borderline' caught on.

An attempt to consolidate the borderline concept into formal diagnosis was made in a paper by Gunderson and Singer (1975). They reviewed the literature and proposed five aspects of diagnosis. The first, labelled affect, included the main affect, anger, as well as depression, anxiety and anhedonia. The second, labelled behaviour, was seen as superficially normal but with less impulse control and often with sexual problems. The third was 'brief psychotic episodes', sometimes with disturbance of consciousness. The fourth aspect was that the sufferer's relationships were seen as superficial. Finally, 'deviant thought processes' were revealed in projective testing.

A comparison of all these models was performed by Perry and Klerman (1978). They noted a number of problems with consistency. Of the 42 items listed across the studies, only one – that the patient's behaviour in the interview is usually adaptive and appropriate – was agreed upon by all four papers. Similarly, no aspect of the personal history of the borderline was agreed upon by all four papers, and only one symptom – brief psychotic episodes – agreed upon by three of the four. Overall, of the total of 104 separate items, around half were present in only one set of diagnostic criteria. The authors, both gifted academics with first class credentials, concluded:

> This apparent lack of agreement over diagnostic criteria has three possible interpretations:
>
> (1) the borderline concept is an illusion; or
>
> (2) the concept is adequately defined by those criteria held in common, the others being nonessential; or
>
> (3) apart from the concept defined by the common criteria, there are subtypes emphasized by different authors.
>
> Although we favor the third interpretation, it is suggested that further speculation await an adequate test of existing diagnostic criteria.
>
> (Perry and Klerman, 1978)

Not surprisingly, the authors suggested one interpretation was the possibility that the concept of borderline is an illusion. More presciently, they suggested that borderline represented the whole range of the psychopathology of personality, suspecting that the diagnosis would have a large overlap with other personality disorder diagnoses. It had been described as a 'character disorder without a particular behavioural speciality' by Mack (1975), somewhat earlier.

If a paper such as this had been published today, this devastating analysis would have been the death knell of the diagnosis. So how did such a vaguely defined and inconsistent syndrome become so prominent and important over the next 40 years? The answer is that it was rescued by the DSM-III Task Force headed by Robert Spitzer, a man with a mission to make diagnosis respectable and reliable. He concluded that borderline, however inchoate and diverse, was important to keep in the diagnostic system.

A seminal paper was published in the *Archives of General Psychiatry* a year later. The APA Task Force on Nomenclature and Statistics decided an effort should be made to develop criteria for one or more of the borderline conditions frequently reported in the literature. Spitzer et al. (1979) noted that members were divided as to the value of such an attempt. The critics pointed out the heavy reliance on metapsychological concepts and the lack of data regarding the validity of the concept. Nevertheless, it was resolved to define the borderline concept operationally in the two ways it was most commonly used. One was the concept of borderline schizophrenia which was called 'schizotypal personality', and the other, the borderline personality, was called 'unstable personality'.

The criteria set for the respective personality disorders were basically developed by expert consensus. For the schizotypal personality items, Spitzer, Endicott and Gibbon consulted with Wender, Kety and Rosenthal, and derived a list of behavioural items using 34 patients, which they then tested on a further 61 cases. For the unstable personality items, Spitzer, Endicott and Gibbon consulted with a 'number of investigators working in the area' and this resulted in more items, which they believed would be adequate to 'tap the key features' (Spitzer et al., 1979).

A questionnaire was developed that contained the two sets of items, plus five additional items thought to be related to the borderline concept, and it was sent to 4,000 APA clinicians. Eight hundred questionnaires were analysed (a 20% response rate). Two-factor analyses revealed two separate dimensions of borderline characteristics, although only a small proportion of the total variance was explained. In addition, the internal consistency revealed only modest support for two separate unitary dimensions. In fact, 54% of the patients met the criteria for *both* schizotypal and unstable personality. Nevertheless, the authors felt that they had demonstrated that it was possible to operationally define two major dimensions in 'borderline patients'. It might be said they found what they were looking for, even though it may not have been there. The name BPD was used because clinicians who had used the concept 'are far from satisfied with the term "unstable PD"' (Spitzer et al., 1979). Borderline personality disorder was therefore recommended and accepted for DSM-III.

So a diagnosis, unrelated to personality research, but arising from mental state abnormalities used to describe the borderline between neurosis and psychosis, became a personality disorder in DSM-III. Not surprisingly, many questions followed, with doubts about both the validity and usefulness of BPD as a formal diagnostic entity. Kroll et al. (1981) investigated the borderline concept in 117 patients and reported that the discrimination between borderline and other personality disorders could not be made. They concluded that the '"borderline disorder" will be a nondiscriminatory synonym for personality disorder' (Kroll et al., 1981). Pope et al. (1983) reported that although BPD could be distinguished from DSM-III schizophrenia and some affective disorders, it could not be separated from histrionic and anti-social personality disorders. In contrast, some researchers claimed BPD could be discriminated from other personality disorders (Barrash et al., 1983; Koenigsberg et al., 1983). The disparate findings were strongly affected by methodological issues.

It has also been speculated whether the introduction of BPD was influenced by clinical and political pressure, particularly that placed by psychoanalysts who felt DSM-III left them neglected (Tyrer, 2009b; Tyrer, 2018b). Despite all these concerns, interest in the nosology and derivation of BPD virtually ended after the mid-1980s. The reasons for this remain uncertain, but two factors certainly influenced the change from natural concerns about diagnostic validity to the clinical prominence of borderline among the personality disorders. The first was that borderline individuals sought treatment in contrast to most individuals diagnosed with other personality disorders. Tyrer has called these groups Type S (treatment seeking) as opposed to the majority, Type R (treatment resisting) who present frequently with other disorders but do not want their personality problems addressed (Tyrer et al., 2003a). The second was that a specific treatment, dialectical behaviour therapy (DBT), was introduced by Marsha Linehan in 1987. Initially, this was a cognitive behavioural form of management of parasuicide (Linehan, 1987b), but it quickly morphed into treatment for BPD (Linehan, 1987a) and the most cited trial (not a very good trial – see Chapter 8) in the history of personality disorder research was published in 1991, reporting on DBT for 'chronically suicidal borderline patients' (Linehan et al., 1991). For clinicians interested in treating personality problems, borderline was the only game in town. Multiple therapies subsequently sprang up, many variations on one or more aspects of Linehan's approach (see Chapter 8) and any concerns about the value of the borderline diagnosis quickly faded.

Concerns about the overlap between borderline and other personality disorders were occasionally voiced. Dahl noted that 97% of hospitalised patients with BPD had another personality disorder (Dahl, 1986); in another large study only 5% of all patients had borderline personality alone (Fyer et al., 1988), and Pfohl et al. (1986) reported only 10% of outpatients diagnosed as borderline did not have another personality disorder. This overlap problem was ignored in most clinical trials by only measuring borderline criteria and ignoring other personality traits or categories. We therefore now have a vast clinical trial literature on treatment for borderline pathology with the majority of patients involved almost certainly having many other diagnoses of personality disorder.

The 1990s and 2000s were the golden era of BPD. The European Society for the Study of Personality Disorders (ESSPD) decided to rename their conference as the International Congress on Borderline Personality since this attracted more delegates. Clinics for borderlines sprang up in public health services as well as the private sector. Cochrane reviews, clinical guidelines and meta-analyses all focused on borderline, and nothing else. By 2008, a review noted that of papers directly concerned with the treatment of personality disorder, close to 90% were specifically about patients with borderline pathology or groups in whom BPD was the predominant diagnosis (Tyrer, 2009b).

Questions about the validity and conceptualisation of BPD re-emerged when the revision of DSM-IV and ICD-10 classifications of personality disorder began. When it was suggested that trait theory offered hope for informing a more scientific classification system, it was difficult to conceptualise the borderline concept as it had not been derived from a traditional personality trait model. Most of the features of BPD are clinical symptoms rather than personality traits, yet all other personality disorders apart from borderline and schizotypal personality disorders are described in terms of traits. Since both of these were derived from the same methodology – in fact, from the same Spitzer study (Spitzer et al., 1979) – this is hardly surprising.

In ICD-11, the equivalent of schizotypal personality disorder is schizotypal disorder. This describes individuals with odd appearances and unusual speech, often with cognitive and perceptual anomalies, and discomfort with interpersonal relationships. Schizotypal disorder is placed among the schizophrenic group of disorders in ICD-11, while in DSM-5 it stays within the personality disorders, and, somewhat bizarrely, is also placed in the schizophrenia spectrum and other psychotic disorders. But borderline (or emotionally unstable, borderline type as it was known in ICD-10) was in the personality disorder section. Borderline personality disorder has only two features – a pattern of unstable and intense personal relationships, and persistent impulsivity, which are in any way trait-based, making it reasonable to conclude that the diagnostic criteria for this personality disorder are out of keeping with other personality disorders (Tyrer, 2009b).

A further problem emerged with both classification committees favouring a dimensional model. This implies that the central features of abnormal personalities should be identifiable in normal personality (albeit to a lesser degree). Arguments over how to best describe normal personality remain, but there is some consensus that the Big Five is a reasonable start. The ICD-11 domain traits map reasonably and predictably onto four out of the five factors. (The openness factor does not seem to be strongly linked with any psychopathology including PD traits.) In ICD-11, dissocial links with low agreeableness, detached with low extraversion, negative affectivity with high neuroticism, disinhibition with low conscientiousness and anankastia with high conscientiousness.

Borderline pathology does not link convincingly with any of the ICD-11 trait domains or any of the Big Five traits. Multiple studies exploring clusters and dimensions have failed to find a BPD personality trait or domain. As Sharp noted, the fundamental problem is that factor analytic studies over the past 20 years have failed to support a categorically defined BPD analysis (Sharp, 2016).

A recent study (Sharp et al., 2015) may help to explain the apparent contradiction that clinicians recognise and treat borderline yet it does not appear to be a distinct disorder. When analysing personality disorder criteria, they reported strong support for a latent factor underlying the nine borderline criteria. However, when the analysis included the other criteria for personality disorder, and a general factor, the borderline symptoms loaded virtually entirely on the general personality disorder factor. There was no specific factor for borderline. In other words, borderline symptoms 'hung together' when examined in isolation but 'disappeared' into a general factor when modelled alongside other personality disorders (Sharp et al., 2015). The most likely explanation is that the borderline criteria capture a general impairment in personality functioning, particularly around self/interpersonal problems (Sharp, 2016). The reason why psychiatric services tend to focus on borderline pathology only are that many of these are Type S (treatment seeking) symptoms and the many Type R symptoms accompanying them are ignored.

Our recent study reinforces this view by showing a strong relationship between BPD symptoms and the overall severity of personality pathology – a correlation of 0.75 (Mulder et al., 2020). This again suggests that borderline symptoms capture overall impairment in personality functioning as defined by the general description of personality disorder severity in ICD-11, but do not constitute a coherent domain or factor.

4.1 Borderline Personality Disorder and Trauma

If BPD symptoms are strongly related to overall personality pathology, then it is not surprising that there is evidence that trauma (particularly sexual abuse) and the development of BPD are associated. However, the strength of this association is inconsistent. A recent review (de Aquino Ferreira et al., 2018) noted that childhood sexual abuse is reported in 16.1% to 85.7% of patients with BPD, depending on the study. This is a wide range, and clearly the aetiological importance of sexual abuse is very different if it is reported in less than one in five patients compared with more than three in four. Similarly, rates of BPD among victims of childhood sexual abuse range from 1.8%, a relatively rare outcome, to 29.3%, a common outcome. One reason for these widely varying estimates may reflect the heterogeneity of the diagnosis of BPD, and the fact that it is closely linked to overall severity of personality disorder. It has been noted, for example, that rates of sexual abuse are less in samples with milder symptoms. It is also of note that while rates of post-traumatic stress disorder (PTSD) in BPD are higher than the general population, some studies have reported that they are similar to other personality disorders (Yen et al., 2002), possibly reflecting the relationship with overall severity. In summary, we can reasonably state that trauma is neither necessary nor sufficient to explain the development of BPD, but it is difficult to go much beyond this somewhat bland statement until we have better designed studies and a better designed diagnosis.

To further complicate matters, a new diagnosis, complex PTSD, has been introduced in ICD-11. For a complex PTSD diagnosis, individuals must fulfil the criteria for PTSD but also have symptoms of disturbances in self-organisation which include the domains of emotional dysregulation, negative self-concept and interpersonal difficulties. The latter disturbances obviously have some overlap with BPD. These concerns about the relationship between complex and standard PTSD, and BPD have led to two recent studies attempting to distinguish the disorders using latent class analysis (Frost et al., 2020; Jowett et al., 2020). Both report that complex PTSD emerged with a distinct symptom profile. There was significant overlap between BPD and complex PTSD, but the symptomatology was distinguishable. There was also overlap between PTSD and BPD, but this was less consistent. In neither studies was a distinct BPD latent class identified.

However, all these findings have not stopped some from arguing that BPD is better conceptualised as a type of complex trauma-based syndrome (Kulkarni, 2017). In some ways this is understandable given the high stigma often associated with the BPD diagnosis (as we discuss in Chapter 9), and the fact that early life trauma is a very important factor in many individuals with this disorder, but at this point, there is insufficient evidence to support such a conceptual change. As we argue throughout this book, dropping the category of BPD and reformulating the symptoms as individual trait-based difficulties which can be helped by specific treatments is likely to improve outcomes more than an exclusive focus on trauma would.

4.2 Conclusion

Borderline personality disorder is conceptually vague, disturbingly defined and has significant practical limitations. It sits, uncomfortably with its schizotypal colleague, neither belonging to personality trait models of disorder, on a rickety fence between neurosis and psychosis, where it often falls off to either side. Both these diagnoses are distinct from all other personality disorders as they are characterised by symptoms rather than personality traits. At least in ICD-11 the schizotypal variant has joined other symptom-based disorders in the schizophrenia section. Unfortunately, as a consequence of political pressure a borderline pattern descriptor or specifier (Tyrer et al., 2019) remains as a lonely and unwelcome visitor to the ICD-11 personality classification. But borderline is a tough old bird and ignores its companions. Similar arguments were made against its inclusion in ICD-10 (Charles Pull, personal communication, 2017), but despite this opposition, it still forced its way in. The same has happened in DSM-5. On the positive side, the idea of borderline personality has been useful in drawing attention to groups of patients with significant pathology, including personality problems, who wished to have treatment and were ignored. However, it has now outlived its usefulness and we now need a more refined and nuanced description of the personality of the heterogeneous group of patients that most treatment studies are based on. To progress with helping individuals with borderline pathology we need to think of borderline, like personality disorder itself, as a spectrum of conditions based on severity (Table 4.1).

The range shown in Table 4.1 illustrates three aspects of borderline; the reason it is so universally described, the 'constancy of inconsistency' and the seductive attraction of making it a diagnosis of personality disorder. Although there are no clear links between borderline and any established set of personality traits, there is no doubt that the triad of unstable mood, erratic relationships and disturbed behaviour are readily identifiable. The inconsistency that is its hallmark makes it different from all other personality groupings but explains how it imprints itself on others and particularly leads to irritation in health professionals. 'Personality disorder: the patients psychiatrists dislike' (Lewis and Appleby, 1988, Chartonas et al., 2017) is not referring to personality disorder as a whole, but to levels 1 and 2 in Table 4.1. If people are unnecessarily challenging, rude and abrupt, it is only too easy to tag the word 'borderline' to the exchanges, even though, on occasions, it may be the professional who is demonstrating the borderline features.

As the severity of the borderline syndrome becomes more pronounced, it spreads ever more strongly into the ambit of personality disorder, and as its presentation is so florid, it is not surprising that it dominates current diagnostic practice. But it does not belong to personality disorder. It is there by default, and just in the same chameleon way its colours fit bipolar disorder, attention deficit hyperactivity disorder (ADHD) and identity disorders, it masquerades as personality disorder also. But it does not belong in the house of personality disorder, it is merely an aggressive and angry lodger.

In 2003, there was a debate about the value of personality disorder at the biennial meeting of the International Society for the Study of Personality Disorders in New York. George Vaillant, an internationally respected psychiatrist, argued against the diagnosis. In the course of this he commented, '70% of the patients attending in our clinics now have a diagnosis of borderline personality disorder. I have a proposition to put to you. Let us stop using the word "patients". Everybody attending the clinics will be called "borderline" until we find an alternative diagnosis after assessment'.

Most of the people at the meeting thought this was a joke, but like all good jokes, it had substance. Borderline personality disorder has all the consistency and value of what our predecessors called 'the vapours', emanations of strange symptoms and behaviour related to emotional hypersensitivity (Gunderson and Lyons-Ruth, 2008) (and thought originally to

Table 4.1 The panoply of borderline

Level of severity	Main description	Characteristics
1	Borderline disposition	Occasional explosions of anger and irritation, inconsistencies in relationships, sudden changes in mood
2	Borderline episodes	As for borderline disposition, but occurring with greater frequency and lasting longer, but not dominating behaviour or relationships
3	Borderline diathesis	A long-standing tendency to be inconsistent in behaviour and mood, with frequent changes in relationships
4	Borderline syndrome	Essentially the same description as borderline personality disorder in the DSM and ICD classifications, representing an amalgam of symptoms and behaviours, including suicidal behaviour, but not influencing other aspects of personality
5	Severe personality disorder with common dominance of disinhibited, dissocial and negative affective domain traits	Borderline features dominate behaviour and so affect all aspects of personality function. Although some would prefer the 'borderline pattern' descriptor here the range of domain traits allows good separation of different groups

be generated in the womb), that merely illustrated mental disturbance. The vapours have much in common with the prejudiced ideas of BPD, being sexist, misogynistic and unflattering, but easily understood as a facet of negative interaction with society. That is where it should remain, as a historical metaphor for distress, not a diagnosis.

Cultural Perspectives
Epidemiology of Personality Disorders

5.1 The Prevalence of Personality Problems

How common are personality problems? The honest, if unsatisfactory, answer is: it depends on your definition. Whether most of us have personality problems, or only relatively few of us, is determined by the context in which the problems are measured. In this chapter, we will attempt to be transparent about how personality problems are defined and measured, and the influence this may have on their frequency. But while acknowledging this, there is more consistency in the epidemiology of personality disorder than in many other aspects of the subject.

We will also discuss measurement of personality problems within their social and cultural context. As we shall see, aspects of personality appear to vary across cultures and this is to be expected as personality depends on interactions. Ways of thinking about our personality are different, and the assumption of the self as an object, separate from the world, located in an inner compartment and comprised of distinct behavioural properties, may not be universal (Fabrega, 1994).

5.2 ICD and DSM Personality Disorder Categories

As discussed in Chapter 1, the history of defined medical entities called 'personality disorders' largely developed in the nineteenth century in Western societies, although it was clearly present in different forms from ancient Greece onwards. We have to acknowledge the cultural boundaries of these descriptions and also to recognise that culture itself can alter the frequency of personality disorder in a population.

It is useful to begin our survey of personality problems by looking at the prevalence rates of personality disorders. Because almost all of these have all been carried out in the recent past, they use the older ICD and DSM categorical diagnoses. Although we argue that they are now redundant and poorly conceptualised, this is still the place to start.

The main studies of national and international prevalence of personality disorders are summarised in Table 5.1. These studies differ with respect to the diagnostic criteria used (e.g. ICD-10 or DSM-III or DSM-IV), measurement (e.g. questionnaires, interviews), sample selection and size. The resulting findings are therefore inconsistent. The first meta-analysis on prevalence rates of personality disorders was published in 2001 and investigated prevalence in 10 community studies; 8 from the USA, 1 from Germany and 1 from Sweden. The notable finding was the high variance of prevalence rates for those meeting criteria for any personality disorder. The rate ranged from 5.9% to 22.5%

Table 5.1 Main studies of national and international prevalence of personality disorders

Date	Authors (journal)	Type of study	Prevalence	Comments
2001	Torgersen et al. (*Arch Gen Psychiatry*)	National (Norway) Oslo only	13.4% overall Avoidant personality disorder the most common	Probable higher rates because study in capital city
2004	Grant et al. (*J Clin Psychiatry*)	National (USA)	14.8% overall Obsessive compulsive disorder the most common (7.9%)	NESARC (US) study prevalences likely to be inflated as level of disability not used in diagnosis (Trull et al., 2010)
2006	Coid et al. (*Br J Psychiatry*)	National (UK)	4.4% overall Cluster A (2%) Cluster B (2%) Cluster C (3.2%)	Before weighting prevalence was 10.7%
2009	Huang et al. (*Br J Psychiatry*)	World	6.1% overall Cluster A (3.6%) Cluster B (1.5%) Cluster C (2.7%)	
2018	Volkert et al. (*Br J Psychiatry*)	Systematic review and meta-analysis	12.2% overall Cluster A (5.5%) Cluster B (3.7%) Cluster C (4.9%)	Western countries only
2020	Winsper et al. (*Br J Psychiatry*)	Systematic review and meta-analysis	7.8% overall Cluster A (3.8%) Cluster B (2.8%) Cluster C (5%)	High-income countries had rates 5% higher than low income countries

with a pooled prevalence of 14% which was somewhat higher than generally believed at that time (Torgersen et al., 2001; Eaton and Greene, 2018).

One statistic that needs to be noted is that the so-called Cluster B personality disorders (antisocial, borderline, narcissistic, histrionic) constitute the smallest cluster in terms of numbers but the largest in terms of society and health service impact. The epidemiology highlights the other personality disorders that are generally neglected by health professionals of all types. This needs emphasis as so many think of personality problems as linked to borderline pathology only.

A second review of community prevalence rates of personality disorders was conducted by Samuels (2011) and included six surveys performed after 2001. The more recent studies were larger and used structured interviews. The pooled prevalence rates across the four studies assessing all 10 personality disorders were more consistent, ranging from 9.0% to 13.4% with a median value of 10.5%.

Two recent systematic reviews and meta-analyses have been undertaken (Table 5.1). One focused on the general adult population in Western countries and reported an overall prevalence rate of 12.16% (Volkert et al., 2018). A more comprehensive global review was published in 2019 (Winsper et al., 2020) and reported a pooled prevalence rate of 7.8%. This lower rate partially reflected the inclusion of low and middle income countries who generally had lower pooled rates than higher income countries; 4.3% versus 9.6%. In summary, the total prevalence rates of personality disorders in Western countries appears to be around 10%. Rates in non-Western countries are around 5% or even lower. Possible reasons for this discrepancy will be discussed in Immigration and Modernisation.

Table 5.2 Summary of global prevalence rates of individual PDs in meta-analyses by Winsper *et al.* (2020) and Volkert *et al.* (2018)

Personality disorder	Pooled prevalence (95% CI)[a]	Pooled prevalence (95% CI)[b]
Paranoid	2.3 (1.6–3.1)	2.1 (0.9–3.8)
Schizoid	1.1 (0.7–1.5)	2.2 (0.2–2.9)
Schizotypal	0.8 (0.5–1.1)	1.5 (0.8–2.4)
Borderline	1.8 (1.2–2.5)	1.2 (0.4–2.3)
Antisocial	1.4 (0.8–2.3)	2.8 (1.8–3.9)
Histrionic	0.6 (0.4–0.9)	0.4 (0.2–0.6)
Narcissistic	1.9 (0.1–5.6)	0.6 (0.2–1.3)
Obsessive compulsive	3.2 (2.4–4.1)	3.2 (1.4. 5.7)
Avoidant	2.7 (1.9–3.7)	2.3 (1.4–3.4)
Dependent	0.8 (0.5–1.3)	0.4 (0.2–0.6)
Any PD	7.8 (6.1–9.5)	11.0 (6.9–16.1)

a Winsper et al. (2020);
b Volkert et al. (2018).

5.3 Individual Personality Disorders

The rates of individual personality disorders are more variable. In the Torgersen study (2001), the most prevalent diagnoses were histrionic, obsessive-compulsive and dependent. The Samuels (2011) study reported that paranoid, obsessive-compulsive and avoidant were most prevalent. The more recent Volkert et al. (2018) study reported that obsessive-compulsive, antisocial and schizotypal were the most common. These results reinforce the idea that although personality disorders have relatively stable prevalence rates when pooling across multiple studies, rank-order prevalence differs. This instability may partially reflect the generally low prevalence rate of individual personality disorders, so allowing sampling error to have a large impact (Eaton and Greene, 2018). Despite this, some patterns emerge: obsessive-compulsive personality disorder is consistently more common; antisocial, schizotypal and avoidant are consistently in the mid-range. Of note is that BPD, by far the most studied personality disorder, is generally lower; seventh in rank in the Samuels (2011) and Volkert et al. (2018) studies at 1.2% and 1.9% respectively.

Table 5.2 summarises the individual personality disorder prevalence rates reported in the two most recent meta-analyses. It can be seen that while individual rates vary, the rank order is reasonably similar. Obsessive compulsive, avoidant and paranoid are most common, with histrionic and dependent the least.

These findings need to be seen in the context of significant limitations. Both recent meta-analyses reported substantial inter-survey heterogeneity among estimates of prevalence. Not only did diagnostic assessments vary, but this variation affected prevalence rates. Studies using two-stage assessments (screening tool then interview) yield significantly lower prevalence rates than one stage assessment (Winsper et al., 2020; Coid et al., 2006).

5.4 Socio-demographic Correlates

5.4.1 Gender

There are consistent gender differences across studies. Men have lower rates of all personality disorders compared to women, with the exception of antisocial, schizoid and narcissistic personality disorders (Eaton and Greene, 2018). Again, measurement may be a limitation. There is evidence of gender bias within personality disorder diagnostic criteria (Jane et al., 2007), leaving the question of whether gender distributions in personality disorder prevalence reflect real gender differences as opposed to biased diagnostic constructs.

5.4.2 Age

Increasing age is thought to be associated with decreased prevalence of personality disorder, especially for Cluster B personality disorders (Samuels et al., 2002), although some studies report higher rates of Cluster A in older age (Seivewright et al., 2002). Again, some of the criteria are associated with age bias which may lead older adults to endorse criteria differently. Since there are few good longitudinal studies (see Chapter 8), these data might also reflect the likelihood that earlier generations might be less likely to have the disorders (cohort effect). In fact, antisocial personality disorder, which has the best longitudinal data, appears to be increasing, at least in North America. Kessler et al. (1994) reported the frequency of antisocial personality disorder has nearly doubled since the Second World War. A similar increase was reported in young adults in the UK (Rutter and Smith, 1995). Additionally, or alternatively, individuals with personality disorder are more likely to die early, with increased rates of suicide, accidents and physical illness, making them less likely to be included in sample due to attrition (Samuels et al., 2002).

5.4.3 Culture and Ethnicity

Until recently, there was very little data on prevalence rates of personality disorders in non-Western, actually non-North American, countries. The recent Winsper et al. (2020) paper supported what many authorities in the area have long suspected; personality disorders are less prevalent in non-Western cultures.

The lower prevalence of personality disorders in low and middle income countries is consistent with findings about personality disorders dating back over 50 years. Most early studies focused on antisocial personality disorder. Although there seems to be a universal or pan-cultural propensity to antisocial behaviour which has been described throughout history and across cultures (Cleckley, 1988), the prevalence of this behaviour varies in different social groups. For example, Murphy (1976) reported that psychopathy was rare in both Inuit and Yoruba peoples. The first study where two cultures could be directly compared used methodology from the Epidemiological Catchment Area Study which reported lifetime prevalence of antisocial personality disorder in Taiwan was around 0.2% compared to nearly 3% in the USA (Compton et al., 1991). Similarly, low rates were reported in a Japanese primary care setting (Sato and Takeichi, 1993). Even with comparable methodologies, it remains uncertain that these data represent actual differences in prevalence. It is possible that Taiwanese and Japanese respondents offered socially desired answers as a consequence of cultural negation of antisocial behaviour (Calliess et al., 2008). However, the fact that higher prevalence was reported in South Korea (Lee et al., 1987), which has similar cultural attitudes to Japan and Taiwan, suggests that there is a real difference in the prevalence of antisocial personality disorder across nations.

The only other personality disorder with reasonable prevalence data is borderline personality disorder. Overall, the studies are similar: borderline personality disorder is globally present but rates vary. A recent review (Neacsiu et al., 2017) reported rates of 0.7–3.9% in adults. They noted a lower prevalence of borderline personality disorder in countries they classified as 'feminine cultures' (e.g. Spain) than in 'masculine cultures' (e.g. USA), and suggested that feminine societies foster emotional expression allowing more opportunities for validation. They also reported higher prevalence of borderline personality disorder in treatment settings in countries they rated as individualistic (9–27%) than those rated as collective (1–8%).

While antisocial personality disorder has been consistently described historically, the clinical features seen in borderline personality disorder were not the basis of formal diagnosis until quite late in the twentieth century (see Chapter 4). Deliberate self-harm was first described with any frequency in the 1960s (Paris and Lis, 2013). Borderline personality disorder may therefore be a disorder of relatively new historical onset recently described in Western cultures. Its spread to non-Western cultures more recently might reflect social contagion. People in low and middle income countries may have changed from expressing distress by somatising or in other forms into expressing it by self-harm.

5.5 Individual vs Collectivism

The countries and cultures where rates of personality disorders appear to be lower include China, Taiwan, Nigeria, Mexico and Japan (Winsper et al., 2020). Not all of them are low income countries but all would be considered collectivist cultures. The individualism–collectivism cultural distinction has been called the most significant culture difference among societies (Triandis, 2001).

This difference in behavioural norms may have some bearing on personality disorder prevalence. The individualism–collectivism model posits that collectivistic cultures are interdependent within in-groups (e.g. family or tribe), shape their behaviour primarily on the basis of in-group norms and behave in a communal way (Mills and Clark, 1982). Their construct of the self, both the expression and the experience of emotions and motives, is significantly shaped by a consideration of the reactions of others (Markus and Kitayama, 1991). Their thoughts, feelings and behaviours are embedded in social contexts (Santos et al., 2017).

In contrast, individualist cultures encourage people to be autonomous and independent from their in-groups. The normative imperative is to become independent from others and to discover and explore one's unique attributes (Johnson, 1985). The construct of self concerns an individual whose behaviour is organised and made meaningful largely by reference to one's own internal thoughts and feelings rather than being shaped by the thoughts and feelings of others (Markus and Kitayama, 1991; Santos et al., 2017).

Plausible consequences of collectivism for personality are readily discerned. In collectivistic cultures group membership is a central aspect of identity and valued personal traits reflect the goals of collectivism. Life satisfaction derives from successfully carrying out social roles and obligations. Restraint in emotional expression, rather than open and direct expression of personal feelings, is likely to be valued since it promotes in-group harmony. Social context and status roles figure prominently in a person's perception and causal reasoning (Oyserman et al., 2002). It has been hypothesised that these strong social control mechanisms may help prevent the progression of externalising and antisocial behaviours.

Plausible consequences of individualism for personality are different. Here creating and maintaining a positive sense of self is a basic endeavour, and having unique or distinctive personal attitudes and opinions is valued and central to self-definition. Individualism implies open emotional expression and striving to attain personal goals. Judgement, reasoning and causal inference are generally orientated towards the person rather than the situation or social context (Oyserman et al., 2002).

Therefore, on the face of it, individualism–collectivism would appear to have a profound influence on the expression, classification and prevalence of personality abnormality in different cultures. Yet there are virtually no studies of the relationship between personality disorders and individualism–collectivism. There is a literature on the measurement of individualism–collectivism in different cultures. Most studies contrast European Americans with other ethnic groups both within North America and across countries. A meta-analysis reported large and stable cross-cultural differences in individualism–collectivism (Oyserman et al., 2002). However, the differences were neither as large nor as systemic as often believed. European Americans were more individualistic and less collectivistic than others. However, they were not more individualistic than African-American or Latino cultures and not less collectivistic than Japanese or Koreans. Only the Chinese show large effects being both less individualistic and more collectivistic (Oyserman et al., 2002).

A revised Hofstede Scale was recently tested in over 50,000 respondents in 56 countries. Again some of the findings are counter intuitive. The most individualistic cultures were Northern European societies, particularly Scandinavian counties and the Netherlands, while the USA was around the middle of the table along with Greece, Portugal and Ireland. As expected the most collectivist cultures were found in Asia and Africa (Minkov et al., 2017). Collectivist cultures emphasise conflict avoidance particularly within in-groups (Minkov et al., 2017). These features are likely to impinge on personality development and expression. There is also evidence that individualism is increasingly linked to socioeconomic development (Santos et al., 2017).

5.6 Social Withdrawal and Individualism–Collectivism

The main domain relating individual-collectivism to personality problems which has received some study is the relationship between social withdrawal or shyness in individualistic and collectivistic cultures. In Western individualistic societies, social withdrawal in adolescents has been found to correlate with poor social and emotional status (Kim et al., 2008). In contrast to data from Western cultures, the data on social withdrawal among Asian collectivistic populations have produced mixed results. Studies have reported that shy Chinese adolescents were not viewed as incompetent but considered well behaved and easily accepted by their peers (Chen and Stevenson, 1995). One study comparing Australian and South Korean students reported that shy and less sociable individuals in Korea showed better social and emotional adjustment than comparable shy Australian students. The authors pointed out that reserved and reticent attitudes are more valued than outspoken behaviour in Korea and that rather than being viewed negatively, shyness is associated with virtues such as courtesy, gentleness and consideration for others (Lee and Oh, 1999). A recent study reported that differences may also be present in the area of self-control with a Chinese sample having higher behavioural self-control than a US one (Li et al., 2018).

Another interesting variant of social withdrawal is the Japanese culture-bound syndrome, *taijin kyofusho*. This term comprises the word for disorder (*sho*), together with fear (*kyofu*), a fear specifically of interpersonal relations (*taijin*). Those who have *taijin kyofusho* could be described as having extreme social anxiety (Hofmann et al., 2010) or, in ICD-11 terminology, as mild, or, more likely, moderate personality disorder with strong representation of detachment and negative affectivity domain traits. Such people, almost all female, are ashamed of their appearance or of their social competence, and often spend years within the confines of their homes without ever venturing outside. A similar condition, *hikikomori*, a form of extreme social withdrawal in adolescents of both sexes, may have the same roots (Teo and Gaw, 2010; Norasakkunkit and Uchida, 2014).

In summary, despite limited data, there is evidence that collectivistic societies protect against some personality disorders. Such societies are likely to promote obligation to groups and punish those who do not promote in-group harmony. There are stricter boundaries around antisocial and externalising behaviours. This hypothesis is supported by the Winsper et al. (2020) prevalence data which reported that the prevalence of Cluster B and Cluster C personality disorders were lower in collectivistic societies, but that Cluster A personality disorders (which it could be argued may be less responsive to cultural and social variables) were not significantly different.

5.7 Personality and Cultural Interactions

Collectivism and individualism may have adaptive advantages or disadvantages in promoting psychological health and well-being. For example, individualism fosters the pursuit of self-actualisation but this may come at the expense of social isolation (Triandis, 2001). Collectivism provides a sense of belonging and social support but may also bring anxiety about not meeting social obligations (Caldwell-Harris and Ayçiçegi, 2006). Within cultures, those who have individualist traits (independent self) value completion, self-reliance and hedonism. Individuals with a collectivist orientation (interdependent self) value tradition, social values and cooperation.

Extreme independence or interdependence might be risk factors for personality pathology regardless of the society individuals finds themselves within. High individualist values, resulting in placing personal goals above group harmony, might underlie antisocial and narcissistic behaviour. This may be particularly so when indulgence and lack of parental control means that children have little practice in impulse control (Cooke, 1996; Li et al., 2018). Similarly, high interdependent values may result in more internalising disorders, such as fearfulness and avoidance, leading to compliant but not innovative adults. Unfortunately, there are no data on the effects of extreme individualistic or collectivistic orientation and its relationship to personality disorders (Caldwell-Harris and Ayçiçegi, 2006).

There are data on the concept of 'person-environment fit'. This suggests that individuals whose characteristics fit well in a given cultural structure tend to show better adaptation than those individuals whose characteristics are different from cultural demands. For example, a comparison of Anglo-American and Mexican-American school children in the US reported that students with the highest self-esteem were independent Anglo-American children and co-operative Mexican-American children (Triandis, 2001).

A study by Caldwell-Harris and Ayçiçegi (2006) contrasted students residing in an individualistic society (Boston, USA) with those in a collectivistic society (Istanbul, Turkey). They reported that in Boston, collectivism scores were positively correlated with social anxiety and dependent personality (as well as depression and obsessive–compulsive disorder). High collectivism scores also correlated with the more positive personality trait of empathy. In contrast, high individualism scores were associated with low self-reports of psychological distress. In Istanbul, a completely different pattern emerged. High individualism scores were correlated with paranoid and narcissistic features, impulsivity, antisocial and borderline personality features. Collectivism was associated with low scores on these scales and less psychological distress (Caldwell-Harris and Ayçiçegi, 2006). These differing patterns of association support the personality–culture clash hypothesis. The idea that individualism is associated with disorders of impulse control (Cooke, 1996; Paris and Lis, 2013) was supported in the Turkish sample but not in the American sample. On the other hand, high collectivism scores were associated with dependence and social anxiety in the American but not in the Turkish sample. Interdependent personality style appears healthier for individuals living in Turkey.

Why a person's individualist or collectivist orientation which clashes with a culture's values is a risk factor for personality pathology or psychiatric syndromes is not clear. Two major possibilities exist. The first is that having a personality which is discrepant from prevailing social values is a stressor leading to peer rejection and punishment by adults. Collectivist orientation in collectivistic cultures may result in positive feelings about accepting in-group norms. Individualistic orientation may result in ambivalence or even bitterness and feelings of estrangement. In contrast, collectivistic orientation in individualistic cultures may result in feelings of personal failure with social withdrawal and low self-esteem. An alternative explanation is that those individuals with a flexible and healthy personality may be more equipped during socialisation and development to internalise cultural values and adapt their style accordingly. Regardless of causality, the personality–culture clash hypothesis appears to have some support and could be seen to extend the 'goodness of fit' model from developmental psychology into the realm of personality and culture.

5.8 Prevalence of Personality Traits across Cultures

The study of normal personality across cultures has received increasing attention over the past decade with non-Western psychologists describing indigenous constructs that resemble individual dimensions or personality traits (Church, 2020). Researchers continue to debate the universality versus cultural uniqueness of trait structure as well as cultural differences in trait measures (Church, 2016).

Most studies use the 'imposed-etic' strategy where researchers transport existing personality measures into new cultural contexts. This work tested the universality of the five-factor model, or 'Big Five' model – comprising traits of Neuroticism, Extraversion, Agreeableness, Conscientiousness and Openness to Experience. These dimensions, which are derived from English personality descriptive terms, have been translated into other languages and measured in different cultural contexts. The traits are also linked to the five ICD-11 domains discussed throughout the book. The studies using the five-factor model generally demonstrated some consistency in different cultures supporting the concept of at least some pan-cultural validity for underlying personality traits (McCrae et al., 1998). However, more recent studies in less educated or preliterate groups such as the Moore in Burkina Faso (Rossier and Rigozzi, 2008) or forager–farmers in Bolivia (Gurven et al., 2013) did not replicate the Big Five, suggesting the universality of such traits may not be as straightforward as initially thought. For example, openness to experience may not be a distinct dimension in Chinese personality structure (Cheung et al., 2003).

5.9 Trait Comparisons

Trait comparison studies have progressed beyond comparisons of mean values of traits in different countries. Church (2016) recently summarised evidence from a range of studies. He reported that European and American cultures are higher in Extraversion and Openness to Experience than Asian and African cultures. Within-country variances are also generally larger in European and American cultures compared to Asian and African ones. Tight cultures (i.e. societies characterised by strong social norms and penalising of deviance from those norms) have higher Conscientiousness and lower Openness to Experience than less tight cultures. The pattern of sex differences in the Big Five domains is generally similar across cultures. Women are perceived as slightly higher than men in Agreeableness, Conscientiousness, Openness to Experience and selected facets of Neuroticism (Löckenhoff et al., 2014).

While trait theorists predict moderate behavioural consistency across cultures, cultural psychologists predict this consistency will be reduced in collectivist and tight cultures, where behaviour is more determined by relationships and situational norms. A meta-analytic review reported that while a consistent self-concept is important for psychological adjustment and well-being in individualistic cultures, it is much less important in collectivistic cultures (Bleidorn and Ködding, 2013). Similarly consistency of behaviour may be less related to well-being, self-authenticity or relationship quality in Asians compared to European Americans (English and Chen, 2011).

Evolutionary psychologists have also supported a personality trait approach to provide an evolutionary perspective on cross-cultural variation. They argue that the universality of underlying traits reflect a fundamental similarity of human interests related to negotiating status hierarchies, affiliations (including sexual partner), perseverance and so forth. Cultures evolving under differing ecological conditions may develop different mean levels of these universal traits. This reflects different contexts for pursuing the universal interests of status and reproduction. Cultures may manipulate the environmental influences to affect the mean level of personality traits so that cultures may differ on which traits are valued most highly (MacDonald, 1998). Individual differences in traits are plausibly attributed to balancing selection processes, whereby different levels of a trait are adaptive under different environmental conditions (Buss and Penke, 2015).

In summary, while there are concerns that measuring personality traits assumes a Western perspective on behavioural classification, there appear to be broadly comparable traits and behaviours across different societies. However, these traits may not be shared by less educated or preliterate cultures. The traits may reflect fundamental human propensities towards survival and reproduction. It seems likely that the expression of these traits and behaviours is shaped by social facilitation and cultural sanctions leading to group differences in their prevalence and manifestations. The larger and better designed studies report the least societal differences and reinforce the idea that personality traits vary more within a culture than across them.

5.10 Immigration and Modernisation: Effects on Prevalence of Personality Disorders

An increasing proportion of the population in Western countries originated from non-Western societies. Studies have reported that immigration is associated with higher rates of mental disorders, such as schizophrenia (Cantor-Graae and Selten, 2005). The association between migration and personality disorders has been poorly researched. The few studies which have contrasted rates of personality disorders in different ethnic groups have generally reported a lower rate of personality disorders among Black and minority ethnic patients compared with White patients (Coid et al., 2006; McGilloway et al., 2010). Studies analysing the relationship between ethnicity and personality disorders in patients presenting at psychiatric emergency services also report a lower incidence of personality disorders in immigrant groups versus indigenous groups (Tyrer et al., 1994; Baleydier et al., 2003; Pascual et al., 2008).

The reason for the lower rate of diagnosis of personality disorders among immigrant groups is uncertain. Most immigrant groups come from traditional collectivistic cultures who may provide rules, values and roles that inhibit emotional expression (so-called "tightness") and have increased community expectations as was discussed previously (Pascual et al., 2008). These cultural practices appear to be associated with lower rates of Cluster B (e.g. antisocial and borderline) personality disorders (Paris and Lis, 2013); the type of individuals most likely to present to psychiatric emergency services and/or found in forensic settings. It may be that as cultures interact, acculturation occurs only in some domains, such as job behaviour and socialising, but not in others, such as religious or family life (Triandis, 2001) so that the protective effects remain. Alternatively, the findings could be influenced by cross-cultural bias, including method bias and item bias. However, most groups reporting the findings believe they reflect genuine lower rates of personality disorder among immigrant groups. It is also possible that immigration is too recent to significantly influence behaviours and comparable or even higher rates of personality disorder may be found in the next generation of families of immigrants.

Modernisation has been defined in a variety of ways but usually includes aspects such as breakdown of traditional roles and values, changes in child rearing patterns, urbanisation and job specialisation. It has been suggested that collectivistic or traditional societies provide members with predictable expectations. Paris (1998, 1994) and Millon (1987), among others, have argued that the breakdown of stable social structures occurring as a result of modernisation creates rapid social change. This instability is said to be a risk factor for psychopathology in general, and personality disorders in particular (Paris and Lis, 2013). It is of interest that high country income status is associated with higher Cluster B (but not Cluster A or Cluster C) personality disorder prevalence estimates (Winsper et al., 2020; Coid et al., 2006).

The primary mechanism by which modernisation affects personality disorders involves the availability of social roles. Collectivistic societies provide relatively secure roles for most individuals. Even vulnerable members of a society have some function which protects them from feeling useless and socially isolated. Their social structures are also less tolerant of deviance and tend to promote behavioural patterns characterised by inhibition and constriction of emotion. In contrast, modern individualistic societies provide less secure social roles with individuals expected to find or create their own. Modernisation rewards active and expressive personality styles and is relatively tolerant of deviance, but may reject individuals who are less autonomous and successful (Paris, 1998).

Most Western societies have experienced accelerating rates of social change over the past 100 years. Rapid social change may replace predictable expectations with more choices. People may face the more stressful task of forging a personal identity without clear models or pathways. Identity formation demands a high level of individualisation and autonomy (Paris, 1998). Parents and society have difficulty transmitting values which appear outmoded; children are encouraged to find their own. These changes may not result in a higher overall prevalence of mental disorders but may influence their form. Paris (1991) suggests that neurotic and somatic symptoms may be diminishing but personality pathology is increasing in modernising societies. High suicide rates in young Inuit males were linked with the breakdown of a traditional way of life and similar findings have been reported across the world (Jilek-Aall, 1988). In an Indian village clinic studied in the 1960s and 1980s, Nandi et al. (1992) reported that conversion symptoms had waned during the past 20 years but suicide attempts were much more frequent.

Finally, we need to consider the export of Western models of personality deviance across the world. A number of cross-cultural researchers have argued that not only are mental disorders based on a questionable model of pan-cultural universality as previously discussed but that the West has aggressively spread this model of mental illness across the world. There is increasing evidence that this has changed the experience of psychological distress in other cultures. The most convincing data on the spread of Western models concern the syndromes of depression, anorexia and post-traumatic stress disorder. There is reason to suspect that syndromes such as personality disorders have been, or will be, similarly exported. The belief that the DSM is a guide to the world's psyche and provides a guide to real illnesses relatively unaffected by culture is presented with similar confidence to those who believed in nineteenth-century Anglo/American/European mental illness descriptions. Only this time the syndromes are spreading well beyond their Western sources.

Some argue that the cultural influence goes beyond the mental illness categories. This may apply particularly to personality disorders where the diagnoses may be seen to introduce core components of Western culture, including a theory of human nature, a definition of personhood and self, and even a source of moral authority (Summerfield, quoted in Watters (2010)). Western culture highly values at least an illusion of self-control and control of circumstances. It therefore strengthens feelings and behaviours that are more changeable and more open to outside influence. The idea that the mind is fragile and that difficult problems of living may be conceived as illness requiring professional intervention (Mulder, 1992; Mulder, 2008) is a largely Western concept. It has been suggested that medicalising ever larger areas of human behaviour and experience is in itself a cultural response, reflecting the loss of older belief systems that once gave meaning and context to mental suffering (Watters, 2010).

5.11 Summary

Personality problems are common. Even the relatively tight definition of traditional categories of personality disorders leads to 1 person in 10 being so diagnosed in Western countries. More loosely defined concepts such as personality difficulty may affect around half the population. In low and middle income countries, the rate of personality disorder categories appears to be lower: around 1 in 20 people. While these estimates of prevalence have significant methodological limitations, the differences do seem to be real. The lower rates in low and middle income countries are mirrored by the fact that emigrants leaving for Western countries continue to have lower rates of personality disorders. Normal personality measures such as the Big Five, while identified the most societies, also have meaningful differences in scores across cultures. These findings are beginning to lead to interest in studying personality disorders and person-ality pathology in different cultures. In particular the individualism–collectivism cultural distinctions appear a promising model to study behavioural differences associated with personality disorders.

Consistent with the model, traditional collectivist (or so-called 'tight') cultures provide rules, values and roles that inhibit externalising behaviour and cultural expression. These practices appear to be associated with lower rates of Cluster B personality disorders and possibly Cluster C personality disorders. In the latter case, it may be that behaviours in Cluster C personality disorders, such as avoidant and dependent personality disorders, are not seen as deviant but as courteous or desirable and therefore not classified as pathological.

In contrast, individualist societies, which encourage people to be autonomous and independent, shape their behaviour by reference to their own internal thoughts and feelings. They have more open emotional expression and strive to attain personal goals. While there may be obvious advantages to such a strategy, there may also be costs manifest in the increased rate of externalising personality disorders.

While these findings are preliminary, they potentially have implications with regard to the development of personality pathology and even suggest possible preventative strategies to reduce the prevalence of personality disorders in the community. The individualist model within modernising societies appears very seductive and may be impossible to reverse even if it were deemed desirable to do so. However, it seems realistic to expect the rate of personality disorders, particularly Cluster B, to continue to increase as modernity continues to break down stable social structures and reduces relatively secure roles for most people.

Chapter

6

Personality and Health

There is a natural curiosity about why some people are healthier than others. One consistent theme is that dispositional variables or personality may predispose people to poor or good health. This idea can be traced back to the writings of ancient scholars such as Hippocrates and Galen who proposed that individual differences in the four humours could predict health outcomes. Galen, for example, warned that melancholic women compared with sanguine women had a higher risk for breast cancer (Van Heck, 1997).

More recently, health psychology has either made, or claimed to find, numerous associations between personality and health. In the 1950s and 1960s, the literature seemed to have character sketches for most chronic diseases. The migrainous patient was described as an emotionally distressed victim of repressed aggression (Adams et al., 1980); the patient with a peptic ulcer as someone with unexplained emotional conflicts (Weiner et al., 1957); and the arthritic patient as shy, emotionally inhibited and socially inactive (Moos and Solomon, 1965). Perhaps the most well-known is the hard driving, aggressive and confronting individuals – the so-called Type A personality – who were postulated to be prone to coronary artery disease and heart attacks. These sketches have become embedded in lay persons' beliefs: workaholics get heart trouble, worriers get ulcers, and those who are too submissive will suffer from headaches (Van Heck, 1997). Despite all these claims, it is now generally accepted that there is insufficient evidence for the view that specific diseases are associated with particular personality characteristics (Friedman and Booth-Kewley, 1987). But the search continues, and as it makes for good stories, it will persist.

6.1 Personality Traits in Relationship to Health

By the 1980s and 1990s, much research (especially from psychology) has focused on personality variation in terms of traits. Trait psychologists have steadily grown in confidence, pushing what was an esoteric subject into the mainstream, so much so that the authors of a well-known book could assert 'traits matter to health professionals, to mental health professionals, to health psychologists, to cognitive psychologists and others. Each of these, it is increasingly obvious, will do disservice to their clients and participants – and then will be acting, advising and experimenting suboptimally – if they ignore trait variation' (Matthews et al., 2009, p. xxvi). As discussed in the other chapters, there is growing consensus among trait psychologists that personality can be described by five basic factors (the Big Five) (McCrae and Costa, 1984). The current labels are neuroticism, extraversion, agreeableness, conscientiousness and openness to experience. These five traits have been linked with a large number of health outcomes. For example, it has been suggested that extraversion helps extend cancer survival times (Spiegel and Kato, 1996).

Conscientiousness, agreeableness and neuroticism have been reported to be linked with health behaviours such as accident control, safe driving and substance risk taking, which may explain part of the association. Perhaps the most striking finding is that conscientiousness is predictive of health and longevity, from childhood through old age (Friedman and Kern, 2014).

Longevity is, for most purposes, the single best measure of health. It is highly reliable and valid, and helps avoid the 'all-cause dilemma' aspect. These are causes where a person has a disease such as cancer but dies of something else. If the study focuses on cancer survival, the death may not be counted even though it is relevant. So the finding that conscientiousness is consistently related to longevity is of some interest. However, repeatedly documenting an association between conscientiousness and longevity contributes little to knowledge without a focus on mechanisms.

For example, a coordinated analysis of 15 longitudinal samples revealed that conscientiousness is the strongest and most consistent personality predictor of mortality (Graham et al., 2017). An individual meta-analysis from seven large cohort studies reported that those in the lowest tertile of conscientiousness had a 37% higher mortality risk compared to those in the highest tertile (Jokela et al., 2013).

There are a number of potential mechanisms linking conscientiousness with longevity with varying degrees of evidence. First, conscientious individuals engage in a variety of important healthier behaviours – they generally smoke less, eat healthier foods, wear seatbelts and take other measures to mitigate risk. Second, they choose healthier environments, maintain healthier relationships and more stable marriages. Third, they are likely to have better careers, more education and higher income. Fourth, such individuals may be more robust and able to mitigate the effects of negative emotions and life events (Friedman and Kern, 2014). A recent larger cohort study of 11,000 individuals tried to assess what aspects of conscientiousness might be important in predicting longevity. They examined the six facets of the trait and reported that a higher propensity to be organised, responsible, compliant with social and moral norms, and hardworking was related to lower mortality risk. Perhaps, surprisingly, self-control was not a significant predictor, while higher traditionalism and virtue was (Stephan et al., 2019).

Research on the five-factor model and health is now so extensive it is difficult to summarise. A recent meta-synthesis by Strickhouser et al. (2017) has attempted to do so. They reviewed 36 meta-analyses which collectively provided 150 meta-analytic effects from over 500,000 participants. The results are interesting: there is a medium-sized relationship between all five factors together and health, suggesting personality is an important predictor of health and well-being. The effect of the five factors is largest for mental health, intermediate for health behaviours and smallest for physical health. This supports those health behaviour models which propose that much of the effects of personality on health are mediated by its effect on health behaviours (Ferguson, 2013). The synthesis also found that conscientiousness, neuroticism and agreeableness were stronger predictors of health than extraversion and openness to experience. This supports previous work of the importance of conscientiousness and neuroticism, but highlights the possibly underappreciated importance of agreeableness; this predicted health almost as much as conscientiousness and neuroticism. These relationships were also stronger in clinical samples.

6.2 Personality Disorders in Relationship to Health

The extensive research into personality traits and health should logically lead to the study of disordered personality and its effect on health. The five factor traits have been credibly linked to personality disorders, particularly in the new ICD-11 classification and the DSM-5 AMPD (Oltmanns and Widiger, 2019). Thus, individuals with low conscientiousness in the disinhibited domain, or low agreeableness, in the dissocial domain, would be predicted to have poor health behaviours and worse physical health together with their mental health problems. Yet, despite the potential interest in this subject, there is only limited research examining the effects of personality disorders, both on physical health in general, and on the physical health of patients with personality disorders.

While a progressing public health agenda in recent decades has anticipated the integration of prevention in both mental and chronic physical health (O'Neil et al., 2015), personality disorder has been largely omitted from the discussions. Despite personality disorder being a potentially influential moderator of the connection between mental and physical health, the link is often ignored (Tyrer et al., 2015). We therefore have very little idea of how common personality disorders are in patients with physical disorders and what their effect may be on the patient's prognosis.

The very limited data available consistently show that personality disorders are common in patients who have chronic physical disorders and that they affect outcome. For example, a recent study reported that 30% of patients admitted to hospital for end-stage heart failure were identified as having a personality disorder and that these patients were more likely to have complex psychiatric and physical comorbidity including alcohol-related causes of cardiomyopathy (Tully and Selkow, 2014). A study on patients with chronic pain and opioid use disorder reported that over half of the patients had a personality disorder (Barry et al., 2016).

Epidemiological research has consistently shown that individuals with chronic pain are more likely to screen positive for personality disorder traits – particularly antisocial and borderline ones (Braden and Sullivan, 2008). High rates of borderline personality disorder (19%) have been reported in chronic pain patients (Campbell et al., 2015).

Personality disorders have also been linked with obesity. High rates of personality disorders (26%) have been reported in obese patients referred for bariatric surgery (Lier et al., 2011). Among those with psychiatric disorders, who generally are more likely to be overweight, those with personality disorders stand out as being particularly obese (Stanley et al., 2013).

What may be more interesting is whether some forms of personality pathology might be associated with better health behaviours and better physical health. The most obvious candidate is the group of individuals within the anankastia domain. Since these patients have higher conscientiousness scores could those with personality difficulty, or even mild personality disorder, have improved physical health? To give an example, a patient with diabetes and personality difficulty in the anankastic domain may be more meticulous in complying with their treatment and so achieve better glucose levels. This potential relationship has never been explored. Most studies have focused on individuals in the dissocial, disinhibited and negative affective domains such as borderline personality disorder or antisocial personality disorder, and find, as expected, these negatively affect physical health.

A good example of the potential impact of personality is a condition called 'brittle diabetes'. People with this condition have frequent admissions to hospital, have difficulty in getting their blood sugar controlled and cause great problems for their physicians. There has long been controversy over the exact nature of this condition, some believing it to be a particular problem of the pharmacokinetics of insulin and others thinking that emotional problems are paramount (Tattersall, 1997). It is only recently that personality status has been examined as a factor. Pelizza and Pupo (2016) compared two groups of 42 patients, one with stable diabetes and the other with brittle diabetes. In most clinical respects the two groups were similar but the brittle group had significantly greater proportions of borderline, histrionic and narcissistic personality disorder.

The other important question is whether treatment of an individual with a personality disorder will improve their physical health. This is particularly important since the elevated mortality begins in younger age groups. Again, there is no evidence. A recent attempt to conduct a systematic review of interventions aimed at improving the cardiovascular health of people diagnosed with personality disorders did not identify any randomised controlled trials. As the authors note, this finding is in contrast to ongoing research into interventions for people with other types of psychiatric disorders, such as psychotic or affective illness (Hall et al., 2019). It appears that, yet again, people with personality disorders are either excluded from trials evaluating physical health in mental health patients or the researchers do not bother to evaluate personality disorder as part of the study.

Given the longevity data and the early onset of personality disorders, we believe that this is magnifying a serious public health problem. We would argue that people with personality disorders are included in trials evaluating the physical health of individuals with mental disorders and that such studies include some measure of personality functioning, since it may be an important predictor of compliance and prognosis.

6.3 Physical Health in Those with Personality Disorders

Looking at the relationship between health and personality disorders in another way, there is increasing evidence that individuals with a personality disorder have higher rates of physical health problems and use a disproportionate amount of health services (Quirk et al., 2015). An Australian survey reported that those identified with probable personality disorder were around twice as likely to have one or more physical health conditions (Jackson and Burgess, 2004). It also appears that having a personality disorder is associated with a reduced life expectancy. A recent study reported that men lose 17.7 years of life and women 18.7 years (Fok et al., 2012). More disturbingly, this elevated mortality was especially pronounced in younger age groups. The causes appear to be both natural, such as elevated physical health problems, and unnatural, such as suicide and alcohol and drug overdoses. But the premature mortality may also be at least partly related to comorbid mental pathology (Yang et al., 2021).

Other studies have reported similar findings. Fok et al. (2014) reported that individuals who endorsed personality disorder screening items were more than twice as likely to report poor health (41.3% vs 15%), and to report having multiple illnesses (19.9% vs 9%). Specifically, these individuals reported higher rates of asthma, rheumatism, migraines and musculoskeletal problems. The British National Survey of Psychiatric Morbidity reported cross-sectional associations between those screening positive for any personality disorder were nearly twice as likely to report having a stroke and one and a half times as likely to have ischaemic heart disease. Importantly, these findings were noted after adjusting for co-variates such as smoking, alcohol and drug use, exercise, socioeconomic status and diabetes

(Moran et al., 2007). Both borderline personality disorder and antisocial personality disorder were associated with increased risk of cardiovascular disease in the National Epidemiological Survey on Alcohol Related Conditions (NESARC). In addition, antisocial personality disorder was associated with increased rates of arthritis, hepatic disease, obesity, diabetes and gastrointestinal disease even after adjusting for multiple confounders (Quirk et al., 2015).

6.4 Conclusion

This chapter raises more questions than it answers. Personality is linked to physical health, albeit less so than to mental health. At least part of this link is due to health behaviours. It is therefore not unexpected that individuals with personality disorders have increased rates of physical health disorders and reduced longevity. It is also well established that in patients with chronic physical illnesses, personality disorders are reasonably common and affect prognosis negatively (with the possible exception of those in the anankastic domain). It is likely that medical conditions which are strongly influenced by health behaviours may have higher rates of personality disorders than those in which health behaviour is less important. But even here the evidence is limited. Rates of personality disorders appear to be high in pain conditions, obesity and alcohol-related cardiomyopathy. However, people with personality disorders also appear to have higher rates of arthritis and cardiovascular disease, even after trying to adjust for health behaviours such as smoking, so the relationships may not be as straightforward as they first appear.

The material in this chapter presents a strong case for physicians to take greater interest in the mental health and personality of their patients, particularly when they appear to present problems in management. The phrase 'parity of esteem' for both mental and physical health could easily be expanded to 'parity of esteem for personality disorders and all health', but it has a considerable distance to go.

It is not as though physicians have been unaware of the importance of this subject; it is just that so few take it to heart in their clinical practice. One of the pioneers of psychological factors in disease was Francis Weld Peabody, a celebrated teacher at Harvard University (where there is still a Francis Weld Peabody Society offering special help to students). In one of his best-known papers he summarised this philosophy:

> Disease in man is never exactly the same as disease in an experimental animal, for in man the disease at once affects and it is affected by what we call the emotional life. Thus the physician who attempts to take care of the patient while he neglects this factor is as unscientific as the investigator who neglects to control all the conditions that may affect his experiment.
>
> (Peabody, 1927, p. 882)

The physician whose shoulders are broad enough to meld physical, mental and personality factors into their patient care is indeed a superlative physician and needs to be honoured as such.

Personality Disorders and Comorbidity with Other Mental Illness

As we have already noted from the history of personality disorder, when very little was known apart from the humoral theory of disease, it was common to think of temperament (aka personality) as the main progenitor of illness, with all other psychological symptoms considered as secondary epiphenomena. For example, Robert Burton described dozens of symptoms linked to the melancholic temperament, rather too many in his view: 'The tower of Babel never yielded such confusion of tongues as the chaos of melancholy doth variety of symptoms' (Burton, 1621; republished 1927).

The idea that personality was intimately linked with psychopathology persisted until at least the middle of the twentieth century. The German school (although it was too disparate to be linked as a unity) of Kraepelin, Bleuler, Kretschmer and others reversed this idea. They absorbed personality problems into the framework of major mental illness so that they now became secondary. Many personality and behavioural abnormalities became understood as variations, or *formes frustes*, of major psychiatric illnesses. So, for example, Kraepelin traced two premorbid personalities, claiming that a cyclothymic disposition was associated with manic–depressive insanity, while an autistic temperament was linked to dementia praecox, a debate that continues to this day (de Lacy & King, 2013). Kretschmer (1922) considered those with cycloid and cyclothymic features (i.e. rapid changes between lower levels of mania and depression) as variants of manic-depressive psychosis. But, despite these suggestions, based mainly on the notion of organic disease, most psychoanalysts regarded personality as the core feature of the psychopathology they attempted to treat (Mulder, 2004).

The suggested association between personality and psychopathology continued to be an active subject in the 1960s and 1970s, particularly in relation to mood disorders. Eysenck claimed psychotic and neurotic depressions were directly related to his psychoticism and neuroticism personality dimensions (Eysenck, 1970). Paykel and colleagues, in a highly influential paper, created a typology based on factor analysis with four categories: anxious depressives, hostile depressives, depressives with personality disorder and a psychotic cluster, and they claimed validation for these subtypes by showing a differential response to amitriptyline (Paykel, 1972). Winokur et al. (1978) introduced the concept of 'depressive spectrum disease' based on the presence of antisocial personality disorder (ASPD), and of alcoholism in first degree relatives. Those without this family history were called 'pure depressive disease'; these types were claimed to influence treatment response. Hagop Akiskal, another highly influential psychiatrist and researcher always buzzing with ideas, suggested as early as 1973 that depression was part of a spectrum with personality abnormality at one extreme and severe depression and bipolar disorder at the other. He and colleagues (1983) later identified a 'character spectrum disorder' based on personality features and lack of abnormal laboratory findings.

7.1 The Impact of DSM-III

As with other models of psychopathology, classification based on an interaction between psychopathology and personality largely ended with the introduction of DSM-III (American Psychiatric Association, 1980). DSM-III separated personality pathology from the now called Axis I disorders such as major depression, panic disorder, alcohol and drug dependence, and eating disorders. Rather than looking at the interaction between personality and other psychopathology, DSM-III took the view that psychiatric syndromes differ mainly in severity and can be separated into homogenous groups based on cross-sectional symptoms.

Although DSM-III acknowledged that psychiatric syndromes can develop in individuals with personality disorders, it suggested that in these cases diagnoses should be made on two different axes: the psychiatric disorder on Axis I and the appropriate personality disorder on Axis II. This is based on the argument, never proven or fully conceptualised, that there is no evidence that personality pathology can be meaningfully linked to Axis I disorders with regard to treatment or prognosis, and simply describing each diagnosis is the best conceptualisation. Most research since then was therefore based on the assumption that the separation between Axis I and Axis II was valid. Although this is convenient and, it could be argued, stimulated research on the treatment of personality disorders, it has led to a simplification of the complex relationship between patient pathology and other psychopathology.

However, Axis II has now been abolished in DSM-5. There are good arguments for retaining a separate axis for personality disorder (Newton-Howes et al., 2015b) as well as for removing it, but the essential point to remember is that they are intimately related. This chapter reviews the evidence for this intimacy and its nature, and also summarises studies on comorbidity between Axis I and Axis II disorders.

7.2 Examples of the Close Relationships between Mental State and Personality Status

We should first clarify the word 'comorbidity'. Comorbidity was defined by Feinstein as 'any distinct additional clinical entity that has existed or that may occur during the clinical course of a patient who has the index disease under study' (Feinstein, 1970). The most important word in this definition is 'distinct'. Comorbid disease is very common, increasing as we get older, so conditions such as arthritis, angina and hiatus hernia commonly coexist but are genuinely independent. The same also applies to some comorbid mental and physical diseases such as bipolar disorder and rheumatoid arthritis.

The main problem with comorbidity in psychiatric disorders is the difficulty in deciding what is genuinely distinct and what is not. As a general rule, largely because of the uncertain state of psychiatric diagnosis, it is best to regard alleged comorbidity as co-occurrence as this does not state any specific relationship between the conditions. You can see from the examples we discuss that it is very difficult to claim complete independence between personality and mental state. (Even though the terms Axis I and Axis II are no longer in circulation, they still remain useful and so are used below.)

7.3 Co-occurrence between Axis I and Axis II Disorders

Co-occurrence is not easy to classify in psychiatry as we have so few independent measures to clarify the nature of any association. It is first necessary to understand the range of possibilities and how they can be interpreted.

7.4 Methodological Issues

There are at least four problems that need to be considered. First, there remain differences about what is meant by personality pathology and the extent to which this differs from personality disorder. While most recent studies have used DSM personality disorder categories, earlier studies often used questionnaires measuring neuroticism or psychoticism, particularly the Eysenck Personality Questionnaire (Eysenck and Eysenck, 1975). Second, as we have repeatedly noted in this book, the validity and utility of the personality disorder categories (in either DSM-5 or ICD-10) is generally considered poor (Livesley et al., 1994; Livesley, 2021). Third, even if one accepts the personality disorder categories, how they are measured significantly affects the rate and type of personality disorder (Zimmerman, 1994). For example, Hunt and Andrews (1992) reported that the chance of having a personality disorder was nine times greater when diagnosed using the Personality Diagnostic Questionnaire than with the Personality Disorder Examination Interview. Hunt and Andrews therefore concluded that the questionnaire was identifying traits only. All the published studies have reported higher rates of personality disorder with questionnaires than with interviews.

Fourth, the psychiatric disorder itself may influence the measurement of a personality disorder. This has been particularly noted in patients with major depression where the description of individual patterns and tendencies are biased by a negative cognitive set. Depressed people are more likely to disclose unflattering characteristics about themselves than with someone who is not depressed (Mulder, 2004). Although it should be noted that some studies have reported that personality disorders measured during depressive episodes are a valid reflection of personality pathology (Morey et al., 2010). Four models have been proposed to explain the relationship.

7.5 Four Concepts of Personality/Mental Illness Relationships

Despite all the problems outlined, no matter how it is measured, there is substantial overlap between personality disorders and psychiatric disorder (see 7.5.1 Personality Disorder and Mood Disorders). The question of how they are related has been conceptualised in a number of ways:

1) *The Vulnerability, or Predisposition Model*: This model refers to the tendency for maladaptive personality traits to predispose an individual to develop a psychiatric condition. The most studied is the link between neuroticism and depression and/or anxiety. But there are many other examples such as antisocial behaviour leading to substance use disorders, or anankastic traits predisposing to anorexia nervosa. These models are popular in theory and research since they offer an aetiological explanation for disorders.

2) *The Complication or Scar Model*: This model describes the development of, or exaggeration in, personality traits as a consequence of psychiatric illness. Examples include early onset chronic or recurrent depression leading to negative affectivity or substance use disorders leading to criminal and antisocial behaviours.

3) *Spectrum or Co-aggregation Model*: This model implies that personality disorders and psychiatric disorders overlap phenomenologically and may reflect vulnerabilities that are simultaneously expressed in the same person. Certain personality disorders are viewed as *formes frustes* of a psychiatric disorder and may result from a common

aetiology. The model has received increasing attention over the past decade using structural models, particularly the Hierarchical Taxonomy of Psychopathology (HiTOP) model. This attempts to address the problems of diagnostic heterogeneity and comorbidity by using a hierarchical dimensional framework (Kotov et al., 2021).

4) *Pathoplasty Model: The Influence of Personality Disorder on the Treatment of Depression and Anxiety*: This model aligns more closely with the DSM conceptualisation of separate personality disorders and psychiatric disorders, but with personality disorders influencing the clinical presentation of the psychiatric disorder, its course and response to treatment. Much recent research has focused on this relationship because of its potential clinical utility.

7.5.1 Personality Disorder and Mood Disorders

The most commonly studied relationship is between personality disorders and mood disorders. A recent meta-analysis reported that around half of patients diagnosed with depression had a co-occurring personality disorder, with a somewhat lower proportion (40%) in those with bipolar disorder. In depression, Cluster A personality disorders were the least common, followed by Cluster B personality disorders, while Cluster C personality disorders occurred most often. In bipolar disorder, Cluster B and C personality disorders had similar rates (Friborg et al., 2014). For individual personality disorders, borderline personality disorder, avoidant personality disorder and dependent personality disorder were the most common in depression, while borderline personality disorder, avoidant personality disorder, dependent personality disorder and paranoid personality disorder were most common in bipolar disorders.

However, the reported variance in studies is very wide with rates as high as 85% in some samples (Friborg et al., 2014). As previously noted, the method of assessing personality disorder was important, with rates being lower when diagnoses were based on structured interviews. Regardless of the exact percentage, co-occurring personality disorders commonly arise in patients with mood disorders (Friborg et al., 2014), and it does not take much insight to note that the personality disorders that are most commonly found also link to the emotions.

7.5.2 Personality Disorder and Anxiety Disorders

Personality disorders are also common in anxiety disorders. Co-occurrence rates range from around 35% in post-traumatic stress disorder (PTSD) to 52% in obsessive-compulsive disorder. Overall, about half the patients with an anxiety disorder have at least one personality disorder. Again, as might be expected, Cluster C personality disorders occur more than twice as commonly as Cluster A or Cluster B personality disorders. The most common individual personality disorder is avoidant personality disorder (anxious personality disorder in ICD-10), and it is particularly strongly associated with social phobia (Friborg et al., 2013).

PTSD is different from other anxiety disorders and might be considered an outlier. It has a lower rate of co-occurring personality disorders with a different profile – more paranoid and borderline personality disorder, together with avoidant and obsessive–compulsive personality disorder. PTSD appears more clinically heterogeneous than other anxiety disorders (Friborg et al., 2014).

7.5.3 Consanguinity: The General Neurotic Syndrome

When two disorders represent two aspects of the same disorder, the word 'consanguinity' is more appropriate than co-occurrence or comorbidity (Tyrer, 1996). The concepts of 'neurosis' and 'neuroticism' have deviated from each other in the last 30 years but still remain very closely linked. The difference is that although neuroticism is still very much in circulation – it is one of the Big Five personalities – neurosis has disappeared following the publication of DSM-III (American Psychiatric Association, 1980). It has been suggested that the two could be brought together as a 'co-axial' diagnosis, the general neurotic syndrome (Tyrer, 1985; Andrews et al., 1990; Andrews, 1996).

The general neurotic syndrome postulates that those who have both anxiety and depressive disorders and personality disturbance in what are commonly called Cluster C disorders are best viewed as a common syndrome. This exemplifies the Vulnerability or Predisposition model of association. The clinical importance of this is that those with the general neurotic syndrome are predicted to have a poorer outcome to standard treatment than those without the syndrome and may be the cause of recurrent depressive and anxiety episodes (Tyrer, 2015). This has been supported by other studies (Dugganet al., 1996; Yang et al., 2021).

Such consanguineous syndromes of personality disorder and clinical symptom groups could be described as Galenic syndromes, as Galen (2019) was the first to link personality status to disease in AD 192. Admittedly, his views about the disease connection were wrong but his descriptions of choleric, melancholic, sanguine and phlegmatic personalities have endured to this day. A Galenic syndrome can be defined as 'a combination of personality disorder and clinical symptom complex so frequently associated that the two conditions should be considered as a single disorder' (Tyrer, 2021). The reader is invited to find others in this chapter.

7.5.4 Personality Disorder and Substance Use Disorder

Data recording the co-occurrence of substance use disorders and personality disorders are less consistent than the mood disorder data. Often the studies look at the rates of personality disorders among individuals seeking treatment for substance use disorders. Two specific personality disorders, antisocial personality disorder and borderline personality disorder, are very frequently reported in those with substance use disorder. Both are associated with higher impulsivity and aggressive behaviour. In individuals with a personality disorder, the risk of a co-occurring substance use disorder is 5-fold for alcohol use disorders, and 12-fold for substance use disorders (Trull et al., 2010). Overall, with a personality disorder, rates of substance use disorders have been reported ranging from 34% to 73% (Verheul et al., 2000). With borderline, the most studied personality disorder, rates of up to 78% lifetime substance use disorder have been reported (Köck and Walter, 2018).

From the perspective of studying patients with substance use disorders, rates of co-occurring personality disorders vary greatly. The rates of co-occurring borderline personality disorder in treatment-seeking patients have ranged from 14% to 72% (Köck and Walter, 2018). High rates of antisocial personality disorder have been consistently reported in patients with substance use disorders, ranging from 14% to 35% in a recent review (Köck and Walter, 2018). Combining the data, about 50% of all people with alcohol use disorders also have a personality disorder (Newton-Howes and Foulds, 2018). Of these, the minority who have detached or schizoid disorders have the best outcome (Griggs and Tyrer, 1981).

In summary, the co-occurrence of personality disorder and substance use disorder is common. This co-occurrence is mainly associated with antisocial and borderline disorders, and is often associated with more severe addiction. Generally, the rates are higher in drug-dependent patients than in those with alcohol dependence.

7.5.5 Personality Disorder and Schizophrenia

There has been very little research into the comorbidity of personality disorders in schizophrenia (Newton-Howes et al., 2008a). As discussed previously, in early descriptions of schizophrenia changes in personality were seen as a fundamental part of the illness course; linked with premorbid predisposition and consequent deterioration over the course of illness. Again, this model was undermined by modern iterations of psychiatric taxonomy leading to the polythetic approach with single diagnoses and multi-morbidity. With this model, prevalence rates of personality disorders in schizophrenia vary widely with an estimated median rate of around 40% (Simonsen and Newton-Howes, 2018). This infers a reasonably strong relationship between schizophrenia and personality disorders. Peralta et al. (1991) have also suggested in a study of 115 patients with schizophrenia that the presence of negative symptoms is highly associated with premorbid schizoid and schizotypal personality traits and disorders. This needs to be replicated.

7.5.6 Personality Disorder and Eating Disorders

The co-occurrence of personality disorders and eating disorders is surprisingly well documented. A recent meta-analysis identified 87 studies from 18 countries (Martinussen et al., 2017). They reported data similar to mood disorders: around half of all eating disordered patients had a personality disorder. There was no difference in overall rates between anorexia nervosa and bulimia nervosa. There was a high prevalence of borderline and avoidant personality disorders in both groups, but obsessive-compulsive personality disorder was more common in anorexia nervosa than in bulimia nervosa (23% vs 12% respectively).

7.5.7 Personality Disorder and Attention Deficit Hyperactivity Disorder

A complicated and sometimes contradictory literature around Attention Deficit Hyperactivity Disorder (ADHD) and personality disorders makes evidence-based estimates of their co-occurrence difficult. Percentages of personality disorder diagnoses in adult ADHD range from 10% to 75%, depending on the sample characteristics. The most common appear to be antisocial personality disorder and borderline personality disorder (Matthies and Philipsen, 2016). A large longitudinal population-based study reported that ADHD was associated with a significantly increased risk of personality disorders with a hazard ratio of 5.8 (Yoshimasu et al., 2012). Prospective studies have linked ADHD in childhood with the development of personality disorders in adulthood (Mannuzza et al., 1991).

7.6 Summary

The fact that all psychiatric disorders have high rates of co-occurrence with personality disorders – usually around 50% – implies that personality disorders, or more accurately, the behaviours encompassed by individual personality disorder categories, are important conceptually, prognostically, and in regard to treatment. However, they are rarely considered during assessment and treatment planning. This, as we will argue, is a major impediment to sophisticated formulation and treatment decision-making in all psychiatric patients. However, the reasons for this neglect are understandable and are strongly related to measurement and conceptual problems.

Despite these problems, there are some findings that are reasonably consistent. The first is that personality disorders are common in patients with psychiatric disorders. Exactly how common is perhaps a surprising revelation. For most major psychiatric disorders, including depression, bipolar disorder, anxiety disorders, eating disorders and schizophrenia, rates of around 40–50% are the best estimate. For other disorders, notably ADHD, PTSD and substance use disorders, the rates are more variable and the precision of any estimate is limited by the modest amount of data. Nevertheless, however they are judged, personality disorders are common, occurring in 30% or more of patients with psychiatric syndromes. In addition, in studies that have looked for it, the co-occurrence appears to be associated with greater severity and poorer psychosocial functioning.

The general neurotic syndrome, the high rates of personality disorder with both substance misuse and groups sometimes described as 'schizoidy' (e.g. high grade autism, Asperger's syndrome and schizotypy) can all be regarded as joint personality disorder and clinical symptom conditions. Perhaps the best name for these groups is Galenic syndromes, as Galen was the first to join up clinical and personality disorder, with all diseases said to be a consequence of the four humours (temperaments), choleric, sanguine, phlegmatic and melancholic.

Despite this high co-occurrence and its probable clinical importance, there is surprisingly little study on the nature of the relationship between personality disorders and psychiatric syndromes. There are also almost no treatment studies that specifically target patients with psychiatric syndromes and co-occurring personality disorders. Most of the studies which have been carried out are in patients with depression. The next section will review the conceptual models discussed earlier which attempt to understand how personality disorders and psychiatric syndromes influence each other.

Vulnerability and Complication Models

Understanding whether personality pathology and complications may cause a psychiatric syndrome is difficult for various reasons. First, there may be an overlap between the symptoms of the psychiatric syndrome and the personality disorder. The most obvious example is between neuroticism and depression and anxiety (see 7.5.3 Consanguinity: The General Neurotic Syndrome). Second, the onset of the psychiatric syndrome may be early so that in older samples, the apparent personality disorder may be a mixture of risk factors and scar effects from the psychiatric syndrome. Third, much of the data is cross-sectional, reporting an association but with little evidence of the direction of causality.

Ideally, assessment of personality before the onset of the psychiatric syndrome would be the best way to deal with the nature of the relationship. Unfortunately this would require a very large pool of subjects. Therefore, much of the data obtained is retrospective. The most studied relationship is between early onset and/or chronic psychiatric syndromes and the rate of personality disorders. The data are inconsistent, for example, earlier studies often reported that early age of onset of depression and anxiety disorders were linked to personality disorders in adulthood. Two recent meta-analyses reported no clear association between age of onset and depression, and that within anxiety disorders, age of onset was only related to social anxiety disorders and Cluster C personality disorders (Friborg et al., 2013; Friborg et al., 2014). Longer duration and chronicity of mood disorders still appear related to high rates of personality disorders (Mulder et al., 2003; Friborg et al., 2014). The mechanism behind such relationships is difficult to elucidate. In many ways it supports a complication (or scar) model in that the depression leads to behaviours associated with a personality disorder.

A further possible interpretation of these findings is that the association may be mediated by risk factors common to both disorders. Kendler et al. (1993), for example, used a genetic epidemiological approach to study the relationship between neuroticism and depression. They reported a strong association but their model suggested that this was largely mediated through genetic factors common to both traits rather than a vulnerability causal pathway. The causal pathway was in the opposite direction; neuroticism was elevated because of the effects of depression (both scar and state).

Substance abuse is often considered secondary to a diagnosis of personality disorder. But common factors, such as difficulties with impulsivity and impulse control, may explain a large part of the co-occurrence. Neuroimaging studies have reported similar findings for patients with personality disorders and substance use disorders, such as reduction in the grey matter in the limbic system (Makris et al., 2008). Similarly, in ADHD, a twin study revealed a high phenotypic correlation between ADHD and borderline personality disorder which suggested a shared, partially common genetic aetiology (Distel et al., 2011). A recent meta-analysis supported the hypothesis that some personality variables are interwoven with ADHD (Gomez and Corr, 2014).

Since we know that environmental conditions are considered important risk factors for personality disorders, any psychiatric syndrome which influences these might be important. The most obvious is parenting style. For example, Ni and Gau (2015) reported that maternal protection interacted significantly with ADHD symptoms to predict a high level of borderline personality disorder symptoms. An interesting question is whether ADHD symptoms influence unfavourable parenting styles; a difficult child may cause a change in parenting style. Similarly, a conduct disordered child might elicit a more punitive parental style which is associated with higher rates of antisocial personality disorder and substance use disorders – a combined genetic and developmental risk (Rosenström et al., 2018).

Spectrum Model

The delineation of the phenomenological relationship between personality disorders and psychiatric syndrome remains confounded by issues of symptom overlap, effect of the psychiatric illness on personality disorder measurement and conceptual issues. One issue which has become clearer is that personality disorders are less pervasive and enduring than commonly believed. This has been acknowledged in ICD-11 by its emphasis on severity and recognising that level of severity may change throughout a person's life.

These changes in severity are particularly relevant in patients undergoing treatment for the psychiatric disorder. In depressed samples there is evidence that treating the disorder often result in an improvement in the personality disorder symptoms. For example, many studies report a significant reduction in personality disorder diagnoses in antidepressant studies (Fava et al., 1994; Mulder et al., 2003). There is consistent evidence that when depressed patients are no longer depressed that their rates of personality disorder are lower (Zimmerman, 1994; Mulder, 2002).

Pathoplasty Model: The Influence of Personality Disorder on the Treatment of Depression and Anxiety

The main evidence that personality influences the course and prognosis of a psychiatric syndrome comes from treatment trials. There seems little doubt that personality traits such as neuroticism, negative emotionality and harm avoidance negatively affect the outcome of treatment for mood and anxiety disorders (Mulder, 2002). The influence of DSM-5 or ICD-10 personality disorder diagnoses on outcome is less consistent but generally reduces the probability of treatment success. The largest meta-analysis reported that the probability of treatment success – whether using antidepressants or psychotherapy – in depressed patients with a co-occurring personality disorder was half that of those without a personality disorder (Newton-Howes et al., 2014). In the UK's Improving Access to Psychological Therapies (IAPT) programme, personality pathology was identified as one of the most significant predictors of poor outcome (Goddard et al., 2015).

A recent review of the effect of personality pathology on the outcome of panic disorder reported an overall negative effect (OR = 2.7) on outcome. The size of the effect was reduced in trials using manualised, standardised psychotherapies or drug treatment (Reich et al., 2018). While the issue seems relatively settled, a new meta-analysis reported no significant difference between individuals with or without a co-occurring personality disorder in terms of depression severity change, response rate and remission rates (van Bronswijk et al., 2020). The authors only included trials using semi-structured interviews and looked at short-term outcome only.

Influence of Personality Disorder on the Treatment of Health Anxiety

There is only one large study that has studied the influence of personality disorder on treatment outcomes for health anxiety and this reported, somewhat surprisingly, a positive effect of personality disorder on outcome (Tyrer et al., 2021). The study was a randomised controlled trial (RCT) of an adapted form of cognitive and behaviour therapy for health anxiety in medical patients compared with standard care in the clinic. Personality status was measured in two ways at baseline assessment: a shortened version of the Personality Assessment Schedule (PAS-Q) and the Dependent Personality Questionnaire (DPQ) (Tyrer et al., 2004a). The intervention was highly effective in reducing health anxiety compared with standard care (Tyrer et al., 2014a), but the most surprising finding was that those with personality disorder showed the largest benefit when comparing the two forms of treatment. This was not a chance finding: those with the more severe personality disorder demonstrated greater differences than those with less severe (Figure 7.1). The assessors in the study had no knowledge of initial personality status when they made their assessments and also, because of the size of the study involving over 400 patients, it is possible to exclude bias in interpreting the results.

The reasons for the better outcome in those with personality disorder (most of whom had strong anxious and anankastic traits) is not fully clear, but in the study those with personality disturbance had lower dropout rates and more attendances for treatment (Tyrer

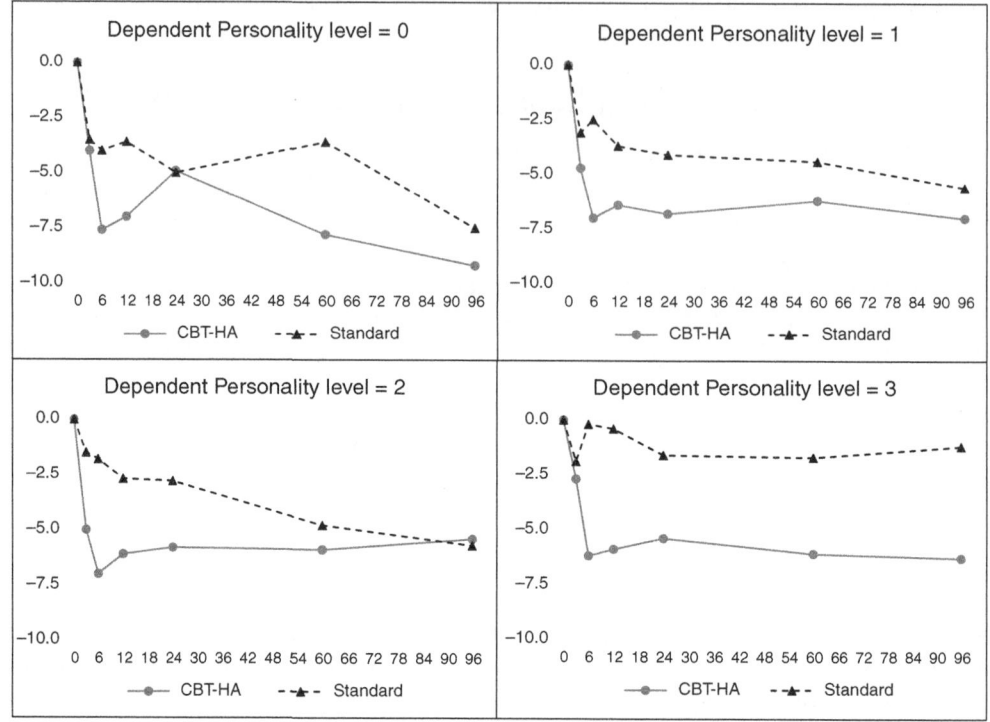

Figure 7.1 Outcome of patients with health anxiety (n=444) randomised to a mean of 6 sessions of treatment with cognitive behaviour therapy or standard clinic treatment separated by degree of dependent personality characteristics, with data recorded over an 8-year period.
(From Tyrer et al., 2021. Reproduced from Personality and Mental Health).

et al., 2021), and this may have been an important factor. As noted in Chapter 6, anankastic domain traits might lead to better health behaviours.

This finding represents a rare positive message for personality disorder. Robert Kendell (1991) concluded after reviewing the status of personality disorder at that time that 'effective treatments for personality disorders would probably have a decisive influence on psychiatrists' attitudes'. Knowing that the presence of personality disorder might be an advantage in selecting treatment is an important step in this direction.

Influence of Personality Disorder on Treatment in Other Syndromes

The influence of personality pathology on the treatment outcome of other psychiatric syndromes is less well studied. In eating disorders, Cluster B personality disorders seem to be related to a poorer outcome in anorexia nervosa and bulimia nervosa, and anankastic traits are associated with a poorer outcome in anorexia (Gaudio and Dakanalis, 2018). Patients with a personality disorder also showed higher rates of dropout. On the other hand, some studies suggest that a co-occurring personality disorder does not influence treatment outcome in bulimia nervosa (Farstad et al., 2016).

The clinical course of substance use disorders appear to be poorer in those with co-occurring personality disorders. In patients with opioid use disorder, the presence of a comorbid personality disorder is linked with increased mortality (Bogdanowicz et al., 2015). Foulds et al. (2017) reported in a systematic review that relapse was associated with higher novelty seeking, reduced reward dependence, lower persistence and cooperativeness. A meta-analysis reported that specific personality traits, notably lack of premeditation and negative urgency, were related to inferior psychotherapy outcomes (Hershberger et al., 2017).

However, Newton-Howes et al. (2017), whose meta-analysis focused on comorbid personality disorders, reported that while patients with personality disorder were more impaired at baseline than non-personality disordered patients with alcohol dependence, they generally shared a similar rate of improvement to that of patients without personality disorder. The only significant difference was that such patients were less likely to complete treatment, which was a reasonably consistent finding across all treatment studies.

There is no empirical evidence to guide the management of comorbid schizophrenia and personality disorders (Simonsen and Newton-Howes, 2018). There is also little data on how personality disorder affects treatment outcome. While personality disorders appear to be common with important clinical implications, most treatments largely focus solely on psychotic elements and rarely address personality pathology, which may then be interpreted as treatment resistance.

Clinical Implications

Given the high prevalence of co-occurring personality disorders in patients with psychiatric syndromes and their largely negative effect on outcome, one might expect that treatment studies would specifically target patients with both disorders. Somewhat surprisingly, there are virtually no studies that have looked at this. While in depression, there is evidence that treating mood symptoms is usually associated with a reduction in personality disorder symptoms (Mulder et al., 2003), there are, to our knowledge, no treatment studies which specifically target these patients by modifying standard treatment. There is some evidence that psychodynamic psychotherapy may improve personality disorder symptoms in depressed patients, even in some where depressive symptoms do not improve (Kool et al., 2003). Higher numbers of psychotherapy sessions may be useful in more complex patients (Van and Kool, 2018), but this has not been systematically investigated.

Three psychotherapies have been developed for the dual disorder of personality disorder and substance use disorders with some evidence from RCTs: modified DBT, dynamic constructive psychotherapy and dual focused schema therapy. Dialectical behaviour therapy was adapted for opioid dependence and borderline personality disorder, and is reported to be more effective than other treatments in female patients (Linehan et al., 2002). Two small RCTs suggest dynamic constructive psychotherapy is effective: the treatment involves weekly individual therapy for 12–18 months. Similarly, two small RCTs reported positive effects for dual focused schema therapy (Köck and Walter, 2018).

Again, to our knowledge, there are no specifically evaluated treatments for anxiety disorders, eating disorders, ADHD or schizophrenia with co-occurring personality disorders.

Summary

The most concerning aspect of this chapter is the paucity of studies examining the interaction between personality and mental illness with regard to treatment. From the few that have been carried out it seems likely that the influence of personality has either been ignored or grossly underestimated. Many more studies, especially longitudinal long-term ones, are needed in this area and it is to be hoped that the forthcoming ICD-11 classification will help to foster these.

Treatment and Outcome of Personality Disorder

Imagine you are a food critic and are visiting a large hotel to evaluate their cuisine. As you are a cook yourself, you first want to visit the kitchens. You are looking forward to the visit as the hotel caters for a large population and is very well appointed. It is a former country house and has many kitchens.

You arrive and are shown into one of the kitchens. There are many cooks, almost too many, bumping into each other, each concentrating on preparing varieties of the same dish. They are all making pizzas: pizza pepperoni, pizza margherita, pizza quattro stagione, mozzarella and basil pizza, and unusual experimental pizzas with mushrooms, multiple cheese pizzas, flatbread pizzas with corn and goat cheese, and sea food pizzas with salmon, shrimps and prawns.

You are quite overwhelmed by the energy and industry of the many cooks, and are looking forward to visiting the other kitchens in the house: 'I'm sorry, but there's not much else going on. Most of the kitchens are empty', says your host. You go into one of them and two cooks, both Dutch, are looking at recipe books and scratching their heads, but they have some interesting ideas. There is another close by, The People's Kitchen. Here visitors can prepare their own food with advice from the chefs and it has attracted considerable interest. But the upgrade in the kitchen is not yet complete and only a limited number can come in.

This is where we are in the treatment of personality disorders. For 'pizza' read 'border-line'. Pizzas are very flexible and can be presented in myriad different ways, but there should be many more dishes on the menu. Hotel Personality Disorder is really only a Pizza Parlour. There are many other potential kitchens but most of them are empty.

8.1 The Pizza Parlour

This analogy is not meant to be frivolous but points out the similarity between the great number of treatments available for borderline personality disorder and so few for others. The preoccupation with a group of dishes that all have the same basic dough and cooking technique is no different from the essentials of the psychotherapy of borderline. The basic structure of the treatment is common, only the toppings are different.

Some might see this analogy as quite unfunny and close to sacrilege. It isn't at all. Two of the major contributors to research into the treatment of personality disorders agree with the premise here. John Gunderson at McLean Hospital in the USA and Anthony Bateman at St Ann's Hospital in London have described the essentials of treatment as good psychiatric management (GPM) (Gunderson et al., 2018) and structured clinical management (SCM) (Bateman and Fonagy, 2009; Bateman and Krawitz, 2013) (Table 8.1).

Table 8.1. Essentials of standard management for borderline personality disorder (and probably all treatment seeking personality disorders)

Good psychiatric management (Gunderson et al., 2018)	Structured clinical management (Bateman and Krawitz, 2013)
• Explain diagnosis	• Reliable appointments
• Be active in therapy	• Assertive follow-up if person does not attend an appointment
• Support via listening, showing interest and selective validation	• Detailed crisis plans
• Focus on 'getting a life' (instead of just on relationships)	• Clear short-term and long-term goals
• The relationship is real and professional	• Group psycho-education and skills sessions
• Change is expected	• Monthly psychiatric reviews
• The patient is accountable, so need to be active collaborators within treatment and taking control of their lives	• Collaborative care plans done together

However you look at these two lists, it is difficult to see how they differ much from good clinical care. People with this condition are a little more sensitive than the average person presenting to services. They sometimes fire off but the therapist should not respond in kind. So a careful planned approach is needed and good boundaries set. Suffering and distress need to be appreciated and acknowledged, and if appointments are missed or crises occur, there needs to be a framework understood by all involved, instead of the angry rejection of 'typical borderline'.

But if you look at any standard text on the treatment of borderline personality disorder, you see a very different pattern (Table 8.2). There is a dizzying range of specialised treatments, all of which have been evaluated in properly designed trials and which appear to offer a dramatic way forward.

More than one of our colleagues have joked that to get on in personality disorder research you need to generate a named treatment for the borderline personality condition, one that can be converted into a three letter acronym, have a guru as its instigator and an

Table 8.2 Tested psychological treatments for borderline personality disorder

Name of treatment	Main proponents	Central feature	Evidence of benefit
Mentalisation-based treatment (MBT)	Anthony Bateman and Peter Fonagy	Mentalisation (mutual understanding of feelings and behaviour)	Bateman and Fonagy, 1999
Dialectical behaviour Therapy (DBT)	Marsha Linehan	Skills training and mindfulness	Linehan, 1987a, 1987b
Transference-focused therapy (TFT)	Otto Kernberg	Self-understanding in relationships	Doering et al., 2010
Schema-focused therapy (SFT)	Jeffery Young	Changing maladaptive patterns of feelings and behaviour	Giesen-Bloo et al., 2006
Cognitive behaviour therapy (CBT)	Aaron (Tim) Beck	Collaborative restructuring of unhelpful beliefs	Davidson et al., 2006
Cognitive analytic therapy (CAT)	Anthony Ryle	Combined CBT and analytic approaches	Chanen et al., 2008
Systems Training for Emotional Predictability and Problem Solving (STEPPS)	Nancee Blum	Combined problem solving and skills-based educational package	Blum et al., 2008
Acceptance and commitment Therapy (ACT)	Robert Zettle	Structured acceptance and mindfulness	Zettle, 2003; Hayes, 2004
Nidotherapy	Peter Tyrer	Environmental manipulation	Tyrer, Sensky, and Mitchard, 2003

expensive published trial showing it is better than doing something a bit less. Only Systems Training for Emotional Predictability and Problem Solving (STEPPS) has bucked the acronym trend. Because of the clear evidence of similarity of models in these different interventions, these are summarised only briefly in the following sections. Good reference texts exist for those who want to follow these up in more detail (Linehan, 1993; Beck et al., 2015; Bateman and Fonagy, 2016).

But the serious point here is that a great deal of effort has gone into developing new treatments for borderline personality disorder that on analysis are no better than mere pizza toppings. This does not mean they are redundant as some people prefer one approach to another, and although all the treatments are lengthy, some are longer than others, but there really are too many.

Gunderson and Bateman have had the courage to examine their preferred approaches and found them to be relatively wanting. These specialised treatments have not delivered quite as much as they promised. This is confirmed by the standard system of meta-analysis, the combining of the results of many controlled trials:

> Findings from randomized controlled trials and meta-analyses suggest that there are several efficacious treatments for borderline personality disorder, including those based on cognitive behaviour theories and psychodynamic theories. In addition, there are generalist and adjunctive approaches. These treatments and the corresponding evidence associated with each are described. It is concluded randomized controlled trials and meta-analyses suggest little to no difference between any active specialty treatments for borderline personality disorder; there are no differences between dialectical behavior therapy and non-dialectical behavior therapy treatments or between cognitive behaviour-based and psychodynamic theory-based treatments. Thus, clinicians are justified in using any of these efficacious treatments.
>
> (Levy et al., 2018)

It is possible that one or more of the treatments described below is demonstrably superior to standard personality management (SPM to add to the three letter acronyms), but as all these studies use classification systems that just give a diagnosis without indicating the severity of the condition, interpretation is difficult. Bateman and Fonagy (2013) are the only investigators to have taken severity into account. They found that structured clinical management and mentalisation-based treatment were similar in efficacy in uncomplicated borderline personality disorder, but when severity (in the broadest sense of including other mental illness) was included the mentalisation-based treatment was superior.

8.2 Brief Summaries of Tested Psychological Treatments for Personality Disorder

8.2.1 Mentalisation-Based Treatment Disorder (Guru: Antony Bateman)

Mentalisation-based treatment (MBT) shares many characteristics with DBT (see next section) but includes more individual and group psychoanalytic therapy. The core element is the somewhat elusive concept of mentalisation, the process that allows us to connect with other people in a way that makes understandable our feelings and those of others. As such it is a central part of our relationships with other people (Bateman and Fonagy, 2016). It also is closely linked to attachment theory and much attention in treatment is paid to the need to develop secure attachments, so often lacking in those with personality disorder.

Mentalisation-based treatment has been evaluated in several controlled trials (Bateman and Fonagy, 1999a; Bateman and Fonagy, 2009; Bateman and Fonagy, 2013; Laurenssen et al., 2018), but its evidence base is still fairly flimsy. Most of the studies have been carried out by the two product champions (Anthony Bateman and Peter Fonagy), and they have been honest enough to explore the treatment with structured clinical management where the differences remain relatively small (Bateman and Fonagy, 2009). But almost all these studies have been carried out with very small numbers, and there is a need at this stage for a large definitive trial including at least 200 patients if two interventions are to be compared. At present the conclusion of Emmelkamp and Meyerbröker (2020, p. 176) is a cogent one: 'It is questionable whether the effects [of MBT] should be attributed to the specific psychodynamic content of the treatment or to the intensive, structured format.' This is an important element to test, not least as much of the support for MBT has come from the psychodynamic community, and it has more recently extended its influence into treating antisocial disorders and those of adolescence (Bateman et al., 2016).

8.2.2 Dialectical Behaviour Therapy (Guru: Marsha Linehan)

Much has been written about dialectical behaviour therapy (DBT) and its use in the treatment of borderline personality disorder. Its originator is a charismatic psychologist, Marsha Linehan, who nowadays would also be called an 'expert by experience', as she developed the treatment for the condition she experienced herself as a young woman when she was repeatedly suicidal. It is a powerful story.

> I was determined to find a therapy that would help suicidal people, people who were deemed beyond saving. I have felt the pain that my clients feel as they wrestle the emotional demons that tear at their souls. I understand what it is like to feel terrible emotional pain, to desperately want to escape by whatever means. Dialectical behavior therapy (DBT) was, and is, my best effort to date at keeping my vow.
>
> (Linehan, 2019)

It is important to understand that at the time Linehan developed this approach, she thought of it as a treatment for severe emotional dysregulation and suicidal behaviour; only later was the focus changed to borderline personality disorder (Linehan, 1987a). The breakthrough for the treatment came with a highly cited paper in the *Archives of General Psychiatry* (a journal which rejected it twice but she kept on persisting, a message for rejected authors everywhere) (Linehan et al., 1991), even though it was not the most impressive of papers, with tiny numbers (see below).

Dialectical behaviour therapy is a combination of treatments including cognitive behaviour therapy, mindfulness and the dialectic of acceptance and change. Because it includes many elements, it is difficult to know which is the most effective and whether any could be discarded. One of the essential elements of DBT is the teaching of new skills, both in group and individual format, and this may be the key ingredient (Barnicot et al., 2016).

Dialectical behaviour therapy is the most frequently recommended treatment for borderline personality disorder by NICE (National Institute for Health and Care Excellence, 2009), and in one of the few studies by independent investigators (i.e. not including product champions of chosen treatments), it was found to be superior to mentalisation-based treatment in terms of self-harm and emotional regulation (Barnicot and Crawford, 2019).

8.2.3 Transference-Focused Therapy (Guru: Otto Kernberg)

Transference-focused therapy is driven by psychoanalysis. It was introduced in principle by Otto Kernberg but developed as a treatment model with the help of Clarkin and Yeomans (Clarkin et al., 1999).

It is difficult to explain transference-focused therapy in a few sentences. It is similar to psychoanalysis in that transference and counter-transference (positive and negative feelings between patient and therapist) are key elements, but, unlike psychoanalysis, it involves the therapist actively. It is based on object relations theory, with patients showing what is termed 'borderline personality organisation' having contradictory internalised representations of self and significant others with strong emotional content that without intervention cannot be accepted together and reconciled. It, like all the other similar therapies, concentrates first on resolving suicidal behaviour before moving on to the emotional contradictory storms.

A randomised controlled trial (RCT) compared transference-focused therapy, DBT and supportive treatment (Clarkin et al., 2007). The results were not striking. All three treatments showed benefits and none was clearly superior to any other. Another study (Doering et al., 2010) with 104 patients gave clearer results. Transference-focused therapy was more effective than treatment from community psychotherapists in reducing suicidal behaviour, admission to hospital and costs.

8.2.4 Schema-Focused Therapy (Guru: Jeffrey Young)

Schema-focused therapy is a mixture of mentalisation-based therapy and cognitive behaviour therapy (CBT), although its devotees would make a strong case for it being quite separate. It combines attachment theory, Gestalt theory, constructivism, psychodynamic concepts and CBT. Because many so-called 'dysfunctional schemata' are formed in childhood a great deal of attention is paid to early life experience, with emphasis on secure attachment (as in MBT), the development of identity and trauma, with particular emphasis on rejection.

The largest evaluation of schema-focused therapy was a randomised trial by Giesen-Bloo et al. (2006) that showed superiority of schema therapy over transference-focused therapy in patients with borderline personality disorder over a three-year period. Suicidal behaviour, compliance with therapy, quality of life and personality pathology were all superior with schema-focused therapy and comparison of the two programmes also showed the schema one was more cost-effective.

But correspondence about this article subsequently pointed out important deficiencies in the study. There was no control group – there really should have been – and the study was helped greatly by schema therapy experts but not by transference-focused ones. It is therefore possible there was some bias influencing the findings in favour of schema therapy (Pearce, 2007; Yeomans, 2007). One of the problems in gathering evidence for complex psychological interventions, especially those carried out over a long time period, is that independent assessment becomes much more difficult. Bias can be generally reduced by both having larger trial numbers with several centres, allowing greater independence of assessments. This particular study only recruited 80 patients.

8.2.5 Cognitive Behaviour Therapy (Guru: Tim Beck)

Cognitive behaviour therapy (CBT) is in danger of being seen as a universal panacea, and this can be a hidden death knell for any treatment as it will eventually overreach and fail. But me-too adventurism does not apply to CBT for personality disorder as this subject has a long pedigree. Aaron Tim (now known mainly as Tim) Beck introduced cognitive therapy for depression in the 1960s and has written about its adaptation for personality disorder for over 30 years (Beck et al., 1990; Beck et al., 2015). Unlike most other therapies, CBT is not just recommended for borderline personality disorder and in his books strong arguments are made for its use in all types of personality disturbance, something from the standpoint of ICD-11 we heartily applaud.

In all personality disorders, the CBT model argues for a longer period of treatment than for symptomatic disorders such as anxiety and depression. This is because the dysfunctional thinking in personality disorder is linked to often-entrenched core beliefs that are more difficult to shift, but the essential principles of treatment follow the standard CBT approach with challenging these dysfunctional beliefs and discovering alternative positive ones. Beck describes this in evolutionary terms as all personality dysfunction (with the probable exception of borderline pathology) has at times in the development of mankind been of some value, so it is not surprising that core beliefs can become ingrained. Beck describes these in terms of strategies, and it is the formerly adaptive but now maladaptive ones that become prominent in personality disorder. So he writes:

> How a situation is evaluated depends, in part, at least, on the relevant underlying beliefs that are embedded in more or less stable structures or 'schemas' that select and synthe-sise incoming data. The psychological sequence progresses then from evaluation to affective and motivational arousal, and finally to selection and implementation of a relevant strategy.
>
> (Beck et al., 2015, pp. 19–20)

The message here is that to concentrate on the immediate symptoms and behaviour in personality disorder is not enough; you have to address the underlying schemas. The most convincing evidence that this is effective comes from the adaptation of CBT in borderline personality disorder from the work of Kate Davidson, a pupil of Beck's, who has written extensively about the CBT approach to both the emotional instability and core beliefs of people with this condition, where it seems to be particularly successful in changing the negative self-image of so many with this condition (Davidson, 2007). Davidson has also carried out important evaluative studies, including a randomised trial with long-term follow-up that showed better outcome than treatment as usual with regard to suicidal thinking and behaviour and also led to cost savings by reduced contact with services (Davidson et al., 2006; Davidson et al., 2010). For those contemplating adapting their knowledge of CBT for personality disorder, it is important to get beyond dysfunctional thoughts. The essential component of therapy is to focus on developing a shared under-standing of the core beliefs about self and others, and then bringing in associated emotions and unhelpful behaviours. Therapy then moves on to strengthening new ways of thinking about self and others and practising more adaptive behaviour.

In other personality disorders there has been less evaluation of CBT. In Beck's latest book (2015), the examples of treatment for each of the named DSM disorders are case examples only, and it is difficult to determine what the specific personality disorder elements are to each of these. Emmelkamp and Meyerbröker (2020) describe the use of CBT in other personality disorders in a useful way for training purposes. Davidson et al. (2009) carried out the first exploratory trial of CBT in 52 patients with antisocial personality disorder and after 12 months found no difference in efficacy compared with treatment as usual, but there were trends in favour of CBT for problematic drinking, social functioning and beliefs about others.

At our present state of knowledge, there is no strong reason for preferring CBT to standard personality management in the treatment of any personality disorder, but CBT skills could still be helpful, particularly in the management of comorbid personality disorder and mental illness (see Chapter 7).

8.2.6 Cognitive Analytic Therapy (Guru: Anthony Ryle)

Cognitive analytic therapy (CAT) is based on an integration of cognitive theory and psychoanalytic object relations theory (Ryle, 1997; Ryle, 2004). It has not been evaluated as fully as CBT but has many strong adherents. It is not a manualised treatment and never can be. The process of treatment has been nicely described as patient and therapist jointly taking up 'a straddling position, with one foot in the therapeutic relationship connecting relationally with the patient and the other foot out of the therapy in an observing position, able to reflect in action on theory, potential ruptures, and enactments in the therapeutic relationship, and on their historical origins' (Ryle and Kellett, 2018, p. 502). Much attention is paid to the role of 'structural dissociation' in the development of separate (reciprocal) self-states, between which patients with borderline presentation can abruptly switch when under stress, in therapy and outside. Cognitive analytic therapy is offered for 8, 16 or 24 sessions, normally of the longer duration for more complex presentations, and with planned follow-up sessions. Early sessions concentrate on a narrative reformulation of the presenting problems and their interpersonal roots, followed by a diagrammatic reformulation. The second of these is a map-like document that is jointly created and used during sessions, and which the patient can refer to quickly whenever unhelpful roles are triggered. Enhanced self-reflection and relational capacity are major aims of therapy.

The most careful evaluation of CAT was a randomised trial published by Chanen et al. (2008), but this showed no superiority over the control condition of 'good clinical care'.

8.2.7 STEPPS (Guru: Nancee Blum)

STEPPS (Systems Training for Emotional Predictability and Problem Solving) is a combined educational and therapeutic training programme focused on the emotional dysregulation of borderline personality disorder (Blum et al., 2008). It is a group treatment delivered over 20 sessions by two trained staff with experience in CBT and basic problem solving. A randomised trial in out-patients showed greater improvements in impulsivity, negative affectivity, mood and global functioning but no difference in suicidal behaviour or hospital admissions (Blum et al., 2008). Although these findings are not particularly impressive, the treatment has strong adherents.

A somewhat similar combined treatment, PEPS therapy (PsychoEducation combined with Problem Solving) was found in a trial of nearly 200 patients with a range of personality disorders to be markedly superior to a waiting list control in terms of problem-solving skills, higher overall social functioning (the primary outcome) and anger expression (Huband et al., 2007). Because of the success of this initial study, a much larger one was planned with over 500 patients with a rigorous design and generous funding from the National Institute of Health Research in the UK. If this had been completed successfully, it would have been the largest clinical trial of personality disorder treatment ever performed. Unfortunately it had to be abandoned early because of adverse effects, including four people who died, two from suicide, in the active treatment group. The treatment was highly structured, with a psycho-education module of up to 4 individual sessions and problem solving of 12 sessions, each of two hours, to improve interpersonal problem skills. A total of 306 patients were randomised, and it is unlikely the results would have been different if the trial had completed its full quota of participants. One of the concerns was that after completion of the interventions, therapy was not gradually tailed off and this may have impacted the final results. One of the few positive results was a saving on total costs (McMurran et al., 2017), but in all cost-effectiveness studies it is difficult to achieve significant differences because of large variation across patients.

The reader may perhaps be puzzled about this account of a negative trial. The reason why we have described it at length is that both authors of this book regard this trial as nearest to the ideal in terms of design and research governance. It set out its aims in a comprehensive trial protocol (McMurran et al., 2011) and had excellent statistical support and expertise, highly qualified economists and good trial supervision. It was also very punctilious in recording adverse events, a process that has been noticed to be rarely carried out with psychological therapies (Duggan et al., 2014). The results were described in coruscating negatives: the treatment was ineffective, it cannot be recommended; there were no buts, no ifs (McMurran et al., 2016; McMurran et al., 2017).

So did this mean the earlier pilot trial, which included very large numbers, was defective as it reported positive results? In one sense it probably was, and if it had not shown good results the big study would not have been undertaken. We think these trials deliver two important messages; it is very difficult to show lasting change in people with personality disorder, and when you use a very rigorous design that largely removes the effect of the personal interaction between patient and therapist, many differences disappear.

8.2.8 Acceptance and Commitment Therapy (Guru: Steven Hayes and Robert Zettle)

Acceptance and commitment therapy (ACT) is the most recent treatment but has not specifically focused on personality disorder but on common symptoms like anxiety and depression. It is sometimes encapsulated in three instructions; wake up, loosen up and step up. So in the first part of treatment the patient is asked to look again at what matters to them in life, rather than incessantly finding ways to prevent or treat their symptoms. The symptoms, or recurrent behaviour, as in personality disorder, are put to one side, and instead all feelings and thoughts are allowed to flow without interruption just as though you were looking at clouds passing overhead on a summer's day. This, of course, is the essence of mindfulness, and is part of DBT.

After this 'wake up' phase, the 'loosen up' phase describes the 'willingness' of accepting any unpleasant feelings, almost as a bystander, so that a better appreciation is made of their status. As Sinclair and Beadman (2016, p. 142) put it: 'it's not about feeling better, but getting better at feeling'. The last phase, stepping up, is the commitment one. The patient is asked to choose which path they want to follow in life and, once decided, they take it. It may involve taking some unpleasant feelings with you, but they should not affect the way that is chosen.

ACT (its inventors say it should be pronounced as one syllable) is described as a contextual behaviour therapy that allows for greater flexibility and is more geared to personal needs (Hayes, 2004; Hayes et al., 2006). We think it is admirably suited to the treatment of some personality disorders, particularly when mood disturbance is a primary feature, but to date there has been only one small trial of its efficacy involving 42 patients with 'borderline symptoms' (Morton et al., 2012). It is an overtly personal therapy that suits the diversity of personality disturbance and could have advantages over other treatments. It is a truly trans-diagnostic intervention that is effective in all forms of mood disturbance (A-Tjak et al., 2015) and also in health anxiety (Hoffmann et al., 2020), where there is considerable personality disturbance (Chapter 7).

8.2.9 Nidotherapy and Social Prescribing (Guru: Peter Tyrer)

Nidotherapy (its first two syllables rhyme with 'Fido') is also trans-diagnostic intervention devoted to changing the environment of those with mental illness (mainly chronic in nature) so a better fit is established between a person and every aspect of their surroundings. It shares some components with acceptance and commitment therapy in that decisions about purpose and meaning in life are addressed, but not attempt is made to change symptoms.

Its theoretical basis is a form of Darwinism. Natural selection leads to organisms prospering when they create a good fit with their environment. In nidotherapy, the aim is to find an environmental fit in terms of physical, social and personal settings that creates an ideal match (Tyrer et al., 2003b). In this context it is worth emphasising that in the original version of *The Origin of Species*, Darwin referred to the 'survival of the adapted', not the 'survival of the fittest'. Although we have been aware of the importance of environment and its effect on mental health for many years, we have usually considered it as something we cannot control and which creates an impact in terms of life events and interactions with genes. But it can also be thought of as a therapeutic tool that can be harnessed for better mental health.

The attraction of nidotherapy in the treatment of personality disorders is that it does not attempt to treat the person, only the environment. This may sound odd, but it does have its focus on the environment – it is not a phony message. The skills of the nidotherapist are in having the imagination to find the best environment and in really good understanding of the psychopathology of the patient so that any suggested changes are matched cleanly (Tyrer and Tyrer, 2018).

Before this is dismissed as nothing new, we need to think about how important the environment is in mental health. Although we all take notice of it, for most it is an issue on the side-lines, and we seldom go about systematically exploring it and thinking of changes that might fit the person in a highly personal and specific way. Once we do this and hit the right environmental changes, all aspects of mental health are improved, even though no attempt has been made to change symptoms or behaviour directly. The other criticism of nidotherapy is that we practise it all the time. We all look for environments that suit our personalities, and once we have found the appropriate niche, we tend to remain in the same ones.

This can reinforce but can also impair adjustment, and if we cut off opportunities for positive change subsequently through lack of courage or awareness, we may suffer in the long term (Roberts and Robins, 2004). This is often the case in chronic mental illness. People become stuck but are too frightened to change; it is called the *Prufrock Syndrome* after T. S. Eliot's famous poem (Tyrer, 2009a; Tyrer and Tyrer, 2018). J. Albert Prufrock is stuck, inactive, watching others live but doing nothing to join them. He says 'there will be time, there will be time' to do all he wants to do, but he remains a permanent watcher, measuring out 'his life in coffee spoons'. Nidotherapy breaks the stuck cycle; it cannot be achieved alone.

Others have recognised the potential importance of environmental change in treating personality disorders (Mordekar and Spence, 2008; Bangash, 2020; Paris, 2020). Social factors cannot be anything other than highly relevant in personality development and its maintenance, so when it comes to management it should not be relegated to the sidelines. As Paris (2020) puts it: 'Social capital remains a missing element: changing cognitions in the present can only be effective if there is a proper environment to apply them.'

The suggestion that the Personality Hotel is too dominated by the Pizza Parlour is not a criticism of the hotel management. Many customers dote on pizzas and will not have anything else, and in the case of personality disorders the same is true. Most of the people who want treatment are in the group of personality disorders called Type S (treatment seeking), the others are Type R (treatment resisting). It may surprise readers to know that most people with personality disorders are Type R; only those with emotional dysregulation and anxiety want to have their personalities changed (Ranger et al., 2009; Gardiner et al., 2010). Nidotherapy is a highly acceptable treatment for Type R personality disorders, delivered in the People's Kitchen at Hotel Personality Disorder. For many in this group an environmental change is the most attractive solution to their problems, sometimes the only one. 'It's not me that's causing problems. It's all those other people – other settings – other restrictions that are the trouble. If you can change those I'll be quite OK.' So while there is no enthusiasm for treatment to change their personalities, important though they might be for others, there is great enthusiasm for changing their life circumstances so that conflict is reduced.

The best evidence for the effectiveness of nidotherapy, an open-ended treatment with no fixed time limits, comes from an RCT of seriously ill patients in an inner city assertive outreach team who had comorbid diagnoses of personality disorder and schizophrenia with many others having substance misuse. Nidotherapy plus assertive treatment was compared with assertive treatment alone. The results showed some clinical benefit in terms of symptomatic change and social functioning but the most prominent change was in costs. Because placements of patients outside hospital were more stable and persisted after discharge, in-patient costs were greatly reduced so the treatment was cost-effective (Ranger et al., 2009; Tyrer et al., 2011b). Although the patients involved had many diagnoses, we felt it was the serious personality disorders that were helped most by therapy.

8.3 Social Prescribing

Social prescribing is a recent addition to the therapies available for personality disorder but it is not promoted as such. It has already been well established that patients with personality disorder consult medical and other health professionals more frequently than other patients and that this is greater for more severe disorders (Moran et al., 2001; Yang et al., 2010). Those with personality disorders are also greatly more likely to incur indirect as well as direct treatment costs so the total cost burden is very high (Soeteman et al., 2008). Any intervention that is going to reduce the strain on primary and secondary care is therefore likely to be embraced enthusiastically by services. Social prescribing is seen by some to be one such intervention. It was introduced in the UK several years ago but only in the last three years has it become a funded part of the National Health Service.

The procedure has been used mainly in primary care for general medical conditions but has now extended to mental illness. There is now a well-oiled procedure in those NHS primary care groupings that are part of the system. Patients who have attended repeatedly and seem to be making no progress are referred to a link worker, a trained professional but not necessarily a health professional, who is well versed in all the facilities in the local area. After assessment, an agreement is made with the patient to make a life change. So the patient undergoing rehabilitation may join a gardening group; the elderly lady with a slow-growing cancer may join a sewing bee; and an arthritic patient with limited movement finds he can get pleasure in a book club.

There is now a National Academy for Social Prescribing but it has yet to launch any significant research. As with many initiatives that on the surface appear to be common sense, researchers have been slow to test its efficacy, its handicaps and adverse effects, its essential and inessential ingredients and its ideal time span. Only qualitative and comparative studies have been published, of generally low quality, with no randomised studies (Bickerdike et al., 2017). Currently most link workers spend up to 12 sessions with their clients. From personal contact it appears that those who have mental health problems are more difficult to assist than others, but it is only recently that the services have taken on this group. There are no data about the proportion of referrals with personality disorders, but it is likely to be high.

It is unlikely to have escaped notice in some places that the environmental changes of social prescribing are very similar to those of nidotherapy and there is much room for exploring these and other environmental therapies together (Tyrer and Boardman, 2020).

8.4 Therapeutic Communities

Fifty years ago the main treatment promoted for personality disorders was the therapeutic community. This all began with what is often called the Northfield Experiments. Northfield is a suburb of Birmingham, and its mental hospital, Hollymoor Hospital, achieved great prominence during the war years when it became a rehabilitation unit for war veterans with neurotic symptoms. This was where the disciplines of the therapeutic community and group psychotherapy were born, essentially as experiments (Bion and Rickman, 1943; Foulkes, 1946; Main, 1946). Faced with many combatants who would probably now be regarded as having post-traumatic stress disorder, they devised a treatment programme involving all patients and staff acting together as potential therapists. Unfortunately, these remained experiments, partly because their essentials were difficult to separate, and though many other units were set up as therapeutic communities, the best known being the Henderson Hospital in Surrey, they have gradually been phased out. In their heyday the writings of Maxwell Jones (1968) and Rapoport (1960) dominated psychotherapy. The principles of democratisation, permissiveness, communalisation and reality confrontation (never properly justified) dominated the fields.

Distinction has to be made between the democratic therapeutic community, where all key decisions are made by the inmates, and the hierarchical, sometimes called concept-based therapeutic community, mainly based in prisons and other correctional institutions. It is a sad reflection on the neglect of research in this area that the first randomised trial of a democratic therapeutic community has only just been carried out, and although this was a small unfunded study, it showed encouraging benefits (Pearce et al., 2017). One of the lasting elements of therapeutic community theory is that patients take a great deal of responsibility in treatment. Any intervention that places responsibility on patients for their progress can be challenging. Pearce and Haigh evoke the principle of 'belongingness' in dealing with potential problems, and this could lie at the heart of successful treatment. Instead of large units like the Henderson Hospital, democratic therapeutic communities are now much smaller and this probably helps communal enterprise and responsibility (Pearce and Haigh, 2008; Haigh and Pearce, 2017).

8.5 Environmental Therapies in Other Settings

In forensic settings, there has been considerable interest in matching the environment to psychosocial management. In the form of management called Psychologically Informed Planned Environments (PIPEs) staff in prisons have been trained to facilitate supportive environments that it is hoped will enable better adjustment on discharge. These promote better exchange between staff and prisoners, more collaboration and the fostering of inter-dependence (Preston, 2015; Benefield et al., 2017). This has not yet extended to treatment after discharge, but the focus on changing environments for the better, promoted energetically by Rex Haigh, now framework lead for Positive Environments at the Royal College of Psychiatrists has been a boost to environmental management in all its forms.

8.6 Psychological Treatment of Other DSM and ICD-10 Personality Disorders

One of the best accounts of treatment of other personality disorders (Emmelkamp and Meyerbröker, 2020, pp. 157–191) describes the evidence for effectiveness of psychological treatments in avoidant and other Cluster C personality disorders, histrionic, narcissistic, antisocial and Cluster A personality disorders (schizoid and schizotypal). These are summarised in Table 8.3.

8.7 Assessment and Treatment of Personality Disorders within the ICD-11 Framework

Because the ICD-11 introduced a radical change in the classification of personality disorders, the findings of previous studies cannot be translated into the new system. Although this might be thought of as a handicap, it is worth reminding all that the treatment studies of individual ICD-10 and DSM personality disorders are rarely of one disorder type as most of them are co-occurring.

So, as described in Chapter 3, the intention with ICD-11 is for clinicians to make a diagnosis of core personality dysfunction in terms of severity (mild, moderate or severe), or as personality difficulty. They then have the option of qualifying the severity levels by describing the behaviours and attitudes, using one or more of the five trait domain traits – negative affectivity, detachment, dissociality, disinhibition and anankastia. Following pressure from researchers in the area, the clinician is also allowed to specify a borderline pattern descriptor or qualifier as an option instead of the domain traits, and this would allow consistency with established treatment manuals. But it is perfectly possible to use the domain traits to define different groups without using the borderline descriptor and its

Table 8.3 Summary of psychological treatments for personality disorders apart from borderline

Personality type	Treatment	Level of evidence	Comment
Cluster A (schizotypal and schizoid)	Modified assertive treatment	Nordentoft et al., 2006 (RCT)	Treatment reduced subsequent development of schizophrenia but personality outcome not recorded
Narcissistic	Compassionate mind training	Gilbert and Procter, 2006	Open study of only six patients with high shame and self-criticism
Histrionic	Vague suggestions only	No published papers	
Antisocial	Cognitive behavioural models and schema therapy	Davidson et al., 2009; NICE, 2009; Koehler et al., 2013; Brazão et al., 2018	Some slight evidence of benefit that is worth pursuing (see text)
Avoidant	Cognitive behaviour therapy and social skills training	Alden and Capreol, 1993; Emmelkamp et al., 2006 (RCT)	CBT better than social skills training and brief dynamic therapy (see text)

retention within ICD-11 remains an anomaly. Our hope is that by having a broader definition and several options of description with the five domain traits the concentration of treatments in the Pizza Parlour described above can be diluted and spread to other dishes.

One of the criticisms of any radical new classification is that it does not allow past evidence to be used in planning treatment. But this is not necessarily true, as the essential building blocks for diagnosis and treatment are already present. We argue that the change in classification will assist clinicians in treating their patients, but of course we have limited evidence of this at present. While all would agree that if we were able to improve the accuracy of clinical description, interventions would be targeted more effectively, with better patient outcomes, at present we have to rely on indirect or proxy evidence.

There are also studies examining face validity and clinical acceptance of the ICD-11 personality disorder classification (Hansen et al., 2019). In addition, the DSM-5 Alternative Model for Personality Disorders (AMPD) is getting increasing traction. This has been widely adopted by researchers and clinicians, and most of the published literature on personality disorders since its introduction has used the AMPD despite it being relegated to 'further study' by the American Psychiatric Association (Mulder and Tyrer, 2019). Fortunately, the ICD-11 and AMPD are largely compatible, at least at the severity and domain trait levels (Bach et al., 2017; Bach and First, 2018).

8.8 Severity as the Diagnostic Criterion in Personality Disorder

Even though severity was not a key component of classification until ICD-11 one of the few consistent themes in the literature on personality disorder is that severity of disorder is the most important single factor in looking at the impact of personality disorder on functioning (Yang et al., 2010; Crawford et al., 2011; Bender et al., 2011; Clark et al., 2018). Both ICD-11 and DSM-5 AMPD (in this chapter, reference to the DSM-5 will use the AMPD, not the official classification) begin their assessment with identifying whether a personality disorder is present and grading its severity as mild, moderate or severe. Both procedures rely on the core capacities of self and/or interpersonal functioning.

The argument giving the central role of severity to the assessment of personality disorder is persuasive. Put simply, it enables clinicians to distinguish those who have the greatest level of personality disturbance from those who do not, and thereby help services target their interventions more effectively. It is also consistent with the evidence that severity, however it is assessed, is associated with higher levels of service contact, more impaired social functioning and higher rates of unemployment (Yang et al., 2010; Crawford et al., 2011). Patients with severe personality disorder have a greater incidence of self-harm, and if they suffer from anxiety or depression are more likely to have a chronic course (Tyrer et al., 2004b). Such patients also suffer more psychosocial impairment (Buer Christensen et al., 2020), have a greater degree of comorbidity and suicide risk (Conway et al., 2016), have lower treatment engagement (Papamalis et al., 2020) and higher risk of treatment dropout (Eurelings-Bontekoe et al., 2009). More recently, evidence suggests that the general features of personality disorder (the so-called 'G' factor, Sharp et al. (2015)) may correspond to a global level of severity. This factor is associated with service use and suicidality (Clark et al., 1997; Conway et al., 2016) and is consistent with research reporting that a global measure of personality functioning outperformed the total categorical personality disorder criteria in explaining psychosocial impairment (Oltmanns and Balsis, 2011).

8.9 Clinical Utility of Severity

As well as helping guide clinicians in deciding who to treat, a general dimension of personality severity may be a good target for intervention and monitoring efficacy. Most psychosocial interventions operate via common mechanisms (Mulder et al., 2017). Schema-focused therapy, for example, attempts to strengthen healthy adult functioning (i.e. a good sense of who one is, a stable sense of self-worth, and appropriate affect and impulse regulation). These goals are trans-diagnostic and apply to all. Similarly, mentalisation-based treatment – where the goal is more about mentalising (the capacity to reflect on one's own and others' mental states) is something all patients with personality disorders would benefit from.

Because a general dimension of personality is changeable, it may be a better way of measuring progress than specific personality traits which are more stable (National Institute for Health and Care Excellence, 2009; Stoffers et al., 2012; Chanen and McCutcheon, 2013). Therefore treatment may improve patients from a severe to a moderate level of personality disturbance (Tyrer et al., 2011a). Higher baseline level of personality disturbance is generally associated with worse treatment outcome. However, patients with severe personality dysfunction may show larger pre-post-treatment effect in terms of improvement. Such patients have more to improve in personality functioning than those with milder personality problems (Bach and Simonsen, 2021), although the most severe personality disorders often show minimal evidence of improvement.

The face value of clinical utility is supported by a recent survey of clinicians which reported that the level of personality function is more useful than specific personality disorder categories when formulating treatments and discussing them with patients (Hansen et al., 2019). Clinicians view the levels of general personality functioning to be associated with prognosis and optimising treatment intensity (Zanarini et al., 2012a) and judged ICD-11 as more useful for treatment planning than ICD-10. In the UK, there is a national service for personality disorder (Royal College of Psychiatrists, 2020; Tyrer, 2020a) in which four tiers of service are described. In selecting patients for each tier severity must be taken into account but is not mentioned in the guidance.

Personality disorder severity is linked to treatment alliance and risk of drop-out (Eurelings-Bontekoe et al., 2009; Papamalis et al., 2020). Perhaps not surprisingly, those with more severe personality dysfunction have lower quality therapeutic relationships and poorer treatment engagement (Soloff, 1998; Kendall et al., 2010). Clinicians also report that more severe personality pathology is associated with boundary confusion, increased negative countertransference and increased need for supportive ventures (Koelen et al., 2012; Gordon et al., 2019). This underscores the importance of assessing accurately the severity of a patient's personality dysfunction and using this information in planning treatment. For example, severe personality disorder may lead towards a more supportive rather than interpretive framework in therapy (Tyrer and Davidson, 2000), or to 'limited reparenting' in a Schema Focused Treatment Model of treatment.

The presence of severe personality disorder should also alert clinicians to carefully monitor their own therapeutic processes since such patients are more likely to induce anger and reduce empathy. Managing this countertransference may be related to better outcomes (Silk and Feurino, 2012). The influence of therapists' effects on treatment outcome may increase with the severity of the patient's pathology (American Psychiatric Association Practice Guidelines, 2001). Greater severity of personality disorder is associated with higher risk for dropout (Herpertz et al., 2007; Lieb et al., 2010) suggesting a more individualised approach to treatment may be necessary. A more cynical approach to care was suggested by Robin (1976) to justify a waiting list for out-patients, using the argument (without data) that those who failed to attend for appointments had 'neurosis or personality problems'.

8.10 Personality Trait Domains

What about trait domains? These present a substantial problem. The vast majority of studies on treatment are in the pizza parlour and as they are labelled as having borderline personality disorder (Storebø et al., 2020), they cross all domains. Factor analytic studies over the past 20 years have failed to support a categorical borderline personality diagnosis (Sharp, 2016) (Chapter 4), and we can say with some confidence that one does not exist. In addition, borderline in all its manifestations does not link successfully with normal personality traits such as the Big Five or any of the ICD-11 trait domain qualifiers (or DSM-5 ones for that matter). There is no specific borderline personality disorder factor (Sharp et al., 2015). So when treating borderline personality disorder, we may be dealing with negative affectivity explained as separation anxiety and unstable mood, dissociality expressed as aggression/hostility, or disinhibition experienced as impulsivity/risk-taking – or, more likely, some combination of these trait domains, possibly with a compulsive element thrown in. The vast majority of individuals fulfilling criteria for borderline personality disorder also fulfil criteria for at least one other personality disorder (Dahl, 1986; Pfohl et al., 1986).

It seems obvious that more focused and meaningful treatments would focus on managing and treating the prominent maladaptive traits rather than a heterogeneous category. Clinicians should treat specific problems (e.g. negative affectivity or disinhibition) rather than diagnoses such as borderline personality disorder (Bach and Presnall-Shvorin, 2020). Personality traits appear to shape our responses to treatment (Bagby et al., 2016) and perhaps, more importantly, appear to be amenable to intervention (Roberts et al., 2017b).

8.11 Assessment of Traits

There are a number of feasible methods of trait domain assessment, but currently there are no official instruments to operationalise the ICD-11 trait descriptions and guidelines. The 17-item Personality Assessment Questionnaire for ICD-11 (PAQ-11) (Kim et al., 2021) is a brief measure that captures the five trait domains. The Personality Inventory for ICD-11 (PiCD) captures the five ICD-11 trait domains and can be administered as a self-report form (Oltmanns and Widiger, 2018) and a clinician- or informant-report form (Bach et al., 2020a). Moreover, the facet-level operationalisation of the PiCD has been developed, which portrays the 5 domains including 20 subfacets (Oltmanns and Widiger, 2020). The Personality Inventory for DSM-5 (PID-5), which has been around for a longer time, measures DSM-5 trait domains but can be used to derive the ICD-11 domains using a simple algorithm (Bach et al., 2017). Recently, the 36-item PID5BF+ has been developed and validated internationally to efficiently capture the combined 6 trait domains of both DSM-5 and ICD-11 including 18 subfacet descriptors (Bach et al., 2020b; Kerber et al., 2020). Perhaps of most relevance to non-research clinicians, the traits can simply be rated based on observations, unstructured questions and other available clinical information (Morey et al., 2013). In considering which instruments to use busy practitioners will be most concerned about their length.

8.12 Treatment of Traits

Traits need to be considered in terms of the personality disposition *and* their related functional impairment. This latter aspect is strongly related to the severity of the personality difficulties. For example, a patient might have prominent features of negative affectivity, which if mild, would lead to some distress in interpersonal relationships, but if severe, could lead to hatred, self-harm and possible dissociation.

The basic clinical principle is that traits tend to be resistant to change, but the level of impairment and adaptations to the traits are less so. It is argued that treatment should target the characteristic adaptation of the patient rather than the traits themselves (Bach and Presnall-Shvorin, 2020). The patient is encouraged to find new adaptive ways of coping with their personality traits. Therapy should therefore focus attention on understanding the traits while attempting to change their consequences. These ideas are not new. Wachtel (1973) suggested that psychotherapeutic interventions should be targeted towards the choices of current environmental stimuli, rather than towards the underlying dispositions. Lasting therapeutic change often depends on modulating the impact of the traits rather than getting rid of them (also see section on nidotherapy).

8.13 Using Patient Traits in the Therapeutic Process

Using traits encourages a collaborative therapeutic approach, which may help promote self-knowledge and insight (Fischer and Finn, 2008). An example is helping patients to identify their own traits and how they are demonstrated in everyday life, then helping them accept that traits are part of their (probably biological) heritage – something that they must own – while conveying the idea that traits can still persist and yet become adaptive. Livesley (2003) suggests presenting the information by discussing the probable adaptive advantages of common traits. This model suggests that the traits themselves are not maladaptive but may become so when individuals have learned to express them in ways that cause dysfunction or may lack flexibility. The focus is not on changing a core part of their identity but rather on specific aspects of behaviour.

Acknowledging the adaptive significance of traits when the context is taken into account may be important. An obvious example is that emotional lability may lead to creativity and artistic excellence. Because traits are context-dependent, they may be valuable in some situations but not in others. For example, the detachment trait domain may be problematic in social situations but useful when cool-headed, self-absorbed behaviour (e.g. an academic researcher or truck driver) is called for. Traits are rarely all or none, but dimensional.

8.14 Using Traits to Focus Treatment

The trait domains seem an obvious way to help focus treatment and this is a fruitful area of further study. For example, patients with negative affectivity as well as disinhibition would usually be considered over-emotional. An important task for therapy, therefore, is to contain this behaviour and attempt to reduce the patient's reactivity by teaching acceptance and better regulation. In contrast, patients with detachment are less emotionally responsive and the therapeutic task is to increase emotional activity while also accepting their trait nature.

As noted above, treatment should focus on modulating trait expressions rather than seeking to change the underlying trait. It should help the patient find more constructive or healthy ways to express the basic trait. The premise is that it is possible to change the expression of maladaptive traits by modifying the environment. Obvious examples are for patients to avoid situations and relationships which evoke negative trait behaviours. An emotionally labile patient may be best advised to reduce contact with those who evoke strong negative emotions as well as apply taught strategies to improve emotional regulation. A detached patient may be best helped by encouraging them to create a way of living that is consistent with their basic stylistic traits and needs, rather than attempting to become even mildly extraverted (Bach and Presnall-Shvorin, 2020).

8.15 Specific ICD-11 Trait Domains

There is currently very little evidence about the usefulness of specific domains guiding treatment. Both the ICD-11 and DSM-5 domains are relatively new. While they are related to the five-factor model (FFM) and despite that model being over 50 years old, there is virtually no evidence on how FFM traits specifically guide treatment and prognosis. Most FFM studies are confined to normal populations. One of the major problems in the field has been this disconnect between personality disorder categories and personality traits. There is also interest in using the so-called 'five spectra' within the hierarchical taxonomy of psychopathology (HiTOP). A recent paper by Mullins-Sweatt et al. (2020) discusses potential treatment interventions for the five spectra: detachment, antagonistic externalising, disinhibited externalising, internalising and thought disorder. These have some overlap with the ICD-11 trait domains, but since they are also recently derived there is a lack of specific evidence about their utility. Nevertheless, we can provide some ideas around the treatment of ICD-11 domains.

8.15.1 Negative Affectivity

This domain is similar to high neuroticism. Negative affectivity is important in that it is strongly associated with treatment seeking and may lead to behaviours, such as emotional crises and suicidal behaviour, which are likely to bring the patient into contact with mental health services. Negative affectivity is associated with increased emotional suffering shared with a wide range of mental disorders as well as physical problems. Because emotional distress is associated with treatment seeking virtually all models of therapy target negative affectivity to some degree (Widiger and Trull, 1992). For example, DBT targets emotional dysregulation (Linehan and Dexter-Mazza, 2008) while ACT focuses on acceptance of negative affect (Hayes, 2004), and MBT attempts to increase emotional regulation with improved mentalising capacity (Bateman and Fonagy, 2016).

As has been noted previously (Bach and Presnall-Shvorin, 2020), the aim of treatment is not to transform a person with high negative affectivity into a carefree and confident individual. Usually the best that can be hoped for is that the patient can better identify and deal with negative automatic appraisals in a healthier manner. Learning better emotional regulation and stress management skills will not convert a patient with high negative affectivity to one with low negative affectivity. But it may significantly improve their tolerance to emotions, thereby helping their mood and anxiety.

A range of emotional disorders share the underlying trait of negative affectivity, and specific, albeit trans-diagnostic, approaches have been developed to help. The Unified Protocol is a cognitive-behaviour approach to mood and anxiety disorders as well as avoidant and borderline personality disorders (Barlow et al., 2011; Sauer-Zavala et al., 2016). The approach targets negative affectivity by reducing stress in response to the experience of strong emotions. The underlying rationale is that reduction of adverse reactions to emotions by improving tolerance leads to less reliance on maladaptive, avoidant emotion-regulating strategies that exacerbate symptoms thereby reducing negative emotions.

Mindfulness-based treatments have also been identified as having value for helping those with negative affectivity cope with challenging life situations (Drake et al., 2017). In practice, patients are encouraged not to judge aspects of negative affectivity as negative but instead to take a gentle, inquisitive attitude which reduces rumination, worry and racing thoughts. Mindfulness is therefore a skill which may reduce the distress associated with negative affectivity. It is part of other psychotherapies including DBT and the Unified Protocol.

Negative affectivity is also substantially related to most maladaptive schemas of emotional disorders as outlined in schema therapy. For example, separation insecurity aligns with the schema of abandonment, while submissiveness aligns with the schema of subjugation (Bach and Bernstein, 2019). Patients with high negative affectivity may benefit from schema therapy, such as enhancement of the patient's healthy adult functions, which protect and sooth the vulnerable part of the patient (Bach and Presnall-Shvorin, 2020).

8.15.2 Detachment

This domain is associated with low extraversion and patients are usually described as a 'loner', shy and with intimacy avoidance. They are unlikely to seek treatment but may feel that they are missing out on life. Sometimes concerned friends or relatives will bring them.

There is little evidence to guide treatment. Behavioural therapy skills training, including approaches such as behavioural activation, might be useful (Lejuez et al., 2011). Possibly more important is to have realistic expectations around what change is possible. This involves understanding the patient and then helping them understand and appreciate themselves (Fischer and Finn, 2008). It is important not to become discouraged by the patient's lack of apparent interest in the therapy; such patients are unlikely to give much positive feedback. The therapist should understand that the low level of positive affectivity is not the same as the patient being shut-down or repressed (Bach and Presnall-Shvorin, 2020). Sometimes changing the environment may be more helpful, consistent with nidotherapy (Tyrer, 2002).

8.15.3 Dissociality

This domain is associated with low agreeableness and includes features such as callousness, manipulativeness, hostility and grandiosity. Such patients tend to be resistant to therapists' efforts to establish rapport, they may be dishonest and will often see other people as the cause of their problems. They may be referred through the justice system or their employer.

It has been suggested that therapists considering treating patients with high levels of dissociality should reflect upon their own ability to confront unpleasant behaviours without moral judgement or defensiveness (Harkness and McNulty, 2006). The therapist should avoid engaging in power struggles or responding defensively when challenged with explicit attempts to share control. Some insight and sensitivity to the patient's worldview may be an advantage.

Treatment goals should be moderate and realistic. There is some evidence that despite resistance to interventions, treatment goals are possible (Ronningstam, 2010; Behary and Dieckman, 2012). A reasonable goal for therapy can be structured around the patient developing an awareness of the costs of using such an antagonistic/dissocial strategy (Livesley, 2003; Harkness and McNulty, 2006). If a reasonable alliance is established, there is some evidence of gains using MBT (Bateman and Fonagy, 2016), schema therapy (Bernstein et al., 2007a) or transference focused therapy (Stern et al., 2017).

8.15.4 Disinhibition

This domain is associated with low conscientiousness. Patients are typically characterised by impulsivity, risk-taking, lack of persistence and irresponsibility. Such patients are often brought to treatment by concerned family members or friends.

Again, there is no evidence-based treatment and few studies even considering this trait domain. The underlying principles of treatment remain similar with the goal is to help the patient live with disinhibition traits (Harkness and McNulty, 2006). Behavioural therapy is an obvious treatment but there are no RCTs. As well as attempting to modify behaviour, the therapist should assist the patient in changing their environment to create an effective reward and punishment system that is naturally maintained in the environment (Bach and Presnall-Shvorin, 2020).

Some have suggested that in clinical settings, disinhibition may be equated with Attention Deficit Hyperactivity Disorder (ADHD), which is consistent with evidence that facets of disinhibition, notably distractibility and impulsivity, capture much of ADHD (Smith and Samuel, 2017; Sellbom et al., 2018). This involves helping the patient find safer and healthier activities that still fit with their need for excitement and novelty.

8.15.5 Anankastia

This domain is associated with high conscientiousness which results in the patient having features of perfectionism, emotional and behavioural constraints, a preoccupation with following rules and meeting obligations, stubbornness and orderliness. Again, such patients are unlikely to present for treatment – seeing the world as particularly disorderly, untidy and morally dissolute.

There are no evidence-based treatments, possibly related to the lack of treatment seeking in anankastic individuals. Again, a logical goal would be to help the patient find more adaptive expressions of their underlying traits, without expectation that the traits themselves would change. It has been suggested that anankastic patients may respond better with specific goals and an active therapist providing direction, guidance and reasonable advice. Being on time is a key component, so consistently referring to a plan within a structured session might be helpful (Bach and Presnall-Shvorin, 2020).

Compassion-focused therapy (Gilbert, 2014) focuses on exchanging self-criticisms (internalised critical/demanding authority) for self-compassion (acceptance and compassion from an internalised 'good' authority). This approach has been suggested as useful (Bach and Presnall-Shvorin, 2020). In addition, modified versions of DBT for obsessive-compulsive personality disorder features and disorder of emotional over-control target the inhibited emotional expression, rigidity and stubbornness characterising anankastic features (Miller and Kraus, 2007; Lynch et al., 2015,). Finally, Sociogenomic Trait Intervention Model has been adapted to a specific treatment approach for problems related to conscientiousness (Roberts et al., 2017a). Again, none of these therapies have been assessed using RCTs.

8.16 Pharmacotherapy

In some ways, the rationale for using drugs in the treatment of personality disorders anticipates the ICD-11 classification. Researchers have largely ignored individual personality disorders and have tried to focus on dimensions of personality pathology. The algorithms generally used to study drug effects were proposed by Siever and Davis (1991) and further developed by Soloff (1998). It proposes four dimensions – affective instability, anxiety–inhibition, cognitive–perceptual disturbances and impulsivity/aggression – that cut across all personality categories, and that drug treatment effects on these dimensions should be studied, rather than individual personality disorders.

It may sound reasonable, but there are two problems; the first is that although this is heuristically appealing, little evidence exists to support the dimensions' validity. They have never been tested in hypothesis-driven studies. The second problem is that although the algorithm was designed to study behaviours across all personality categories, over 70% of all field trials involve patients with borderline personality disorder. In addition, most trials are greatly underpowered with a mean of 22.4 participants in one treatment group, and 19.3 in the control group (Duggan et al., 2008). The general recommendation for the numbers needed to test an intervention adequately in an RCT in psychiatry is 100 in each arm of the trial (Johnson, 1998).

Perhaps not surprisingly, recommendations about drug treatment are confusing and, at times, contradictory. The treatment guidelines all focus on borderline personality disorder. Since samples of individuals with this disorder are heterogeneous, the results are bound to be inconsistent. Some guidelines advocate symptom targeted pharmacotherapy based on Siever and Davis's dimensions while others state drug treatment should generally be avoided in patients with borderline personality disorder.

The APA guideline (American Psychiatric Association Practice Guidelines, 2001) stated boldly, without good reason, that symptom-targeted pharmacotherapy was an important adjunctive treatment. They suggest that affective instability is treated with SSRIs (selective serotonin reuptake inhibitors) or MAOIs (monoamine oxidase inhibitors), impulsive aggression with SSRIs or mood stabilisers, and cognitive-perceptual disturbances treated with low dose antipsychotics. The World Federation of Societies of Biological Psychiatry guidelines (Herpertz et al., 2007) state that moderate evidence exists for antipsychotic drugs being effective for cognitive–perceptual and impulsive–aggressive symptoms; that some evidence exists for SSRIs being effective for emotional dysregulation; and that there is some evidence for mood stabilisers being effective for emotional dysregulation and impulsive–aggressive symptoms. The most recent Cochrane Review (Lieb et al., 2010) partially contradicted these guidelines reporting no evidence for the efficacy of SSRIs but did report that mood stabilisers could diminish affective dysregulation and impulsive–aggressive symptoms in patients with borderline personality disorder and that anti-psychotics could improve cognitive–perceptual symptoms and affective dysregulation.

In contrast, the UK NICE guidelines (National Institute for Health and Care Excellence, 2009) state that drug treatment should generally be avoided, except in a crisis, and then given for no longer than one week. There was also concern expressed in the NICE guideline group that at least some of the trials of effective treatments were fraudulent, but as the data from them could not be obtained no definite conclusions could be drawn. The strongest evidence in the published literature came from the use of mood stabilisers. This was tested with lamotrigine (one of the few mood stabilisers that can be used in patients who might become pregnant), in a large trial supported by the National Institute of Health Research, but it reported no benefit for lamotrigine compared with placebo (Crawford et al., 2018). The more recent guidelines for treatment of borderline personality disorder from the Australian National Health and Medical Research Council (NHMRC) (National Health and Medical Research Council, 2012) again reviewed the literature including conducting a series of meta-analyses. They concluded that pharmacotherapy did not appear to be effective in altering the nature and course of borderline personality disorder.

These apparently contradictory recommendations may reflect the weight given to risks as well as benefits of drug treatment. Both the NICE and NHMRC Committees acknowledged that evidence existed that some second generation antipsychotics (notably aripiprazole and olanzapine) and mood stabilisers (notably topiramate, lamotrigine and valproate) may reduce borderline personality disorder symptoms over the short term. They concluded that the substantial long-term risks did not justify recommending these drugs when alternative psychosocial interventions do not carry such risks.

A pragmatic compromise may be to acknowledge the real concerns about using drugs in this population and be guided towards using drugs with at least some evidence of efficacy, using them sparingly and for short periods. The current evidence, from 12 years ago (Abraham and Calabrese, 2008) suggested using atypical antipsychotics and mood stabilisers rather than SSRIs (but see Crawford et al. (2018)), tricyclic antidepressants and benzodiazepines, and more radical therapies to counteract the effects of trauma have also been suggested (Olabi and Hall, 2010). A more radical view, articulated in the NICE guidelines (National Institute for Health and Care Excellence, 2009), is that if patients have no comorbid illness, efforts should be made to reduce or stop pharmacotherapy.

The ICD-11 domain structure would, on the face of it, appear a more promising model than the ICD-10 or DSM-5 models, to test the effects of drugs on personality disorders. The domains may, at least theoretically, be related to drug effects. The disinhibited domain might benefit from atypical antipsychotics or possibly mood stabilisers. Increased negative affectivity might respond, at least partially, to anti-depressant and anti-anxiety drugs. It is possible that agents with anti-obsessive properties, such as serotonergic antidepressants, might help reduce anankastic behaviours. It seems unlikely that medication would have much effect on dissociality given the lack of evidence that they have any effect on antisocial personality disorder (Duggan et al., 2008; Khalifa et al., 2010). There have been no drug studies on patients with detached or schizoid personality traits. Whether drugs ever justify their long-term risk in patients with personality disorders remains contentious. However, the ICD-11 model offers a more plausible and coherent model to test out their efficacy in the short and long term.

In interpreting the data on drug treatment we also have to be aware that anxiety and depression, in all its forms, are found in patients with borderline personality disorder, so any improvement may be a consequence of successful treatment of these other conditions.

8.17 Patients with Multiple Traits

While we have focused on treatment and single personality domains for illustrative purposes, this is a simplistic approach. Many patients will have more than one trait domain affected, particularly if they have moderate or severe personality disorder. A more finely detailed formulation is appropriate for these patients. Some years ago a personality profile of Adolf Hitler was created with the help of psycho-historians. In ICD-11 terms Hitler would have scored highly on dissocial, disinhibited, negative affective and anankastic traits (Henry et al., 1993). Dealing with these would have challenged even the best of therapists and any attempt to portray Hitler as a cooperative patient would be stretching reality.

In another example, two patients in whom negative affectivity constitutes the most prominent feature but one has a secondary trait of disinhibition and the other a secondary domain of detachment. In the former, the behaviour exhibited is externalising anger or overcompensating grandiosity related to dysregulated emotion, while the latter presents with internalising features of withdrawal, depression-proneness and anxiety. Obviously the secondary traits have substantial consequences for treatment planning and targets.

Traditional personality disorder categories are often composed of different constellations of overlapping trait domains. For example, a constellation of dissocial and disinhibition captures much of antisocial personality disorder (Bateman and Fonagy, 2016), while negative affectivity and detachment capture much of avoidant personality disorder. While pure anankastia is similar to obsessive–compulsive personality disorder (Simon, 2015), when associated with negative affectivity, it may be treated as a conscientious and worried type, while when associated with dissociality, it may be treated as a bureaucratic and narcissistic type (Bach and Presnall-Shvorin, 2020). Borderline personality disorder is the most heterogeneous and complex personality disorder and is usually comprised of different domains. Milder cases may largely be characterised primarily by negative affectivity; anxiousness, separation anxiety and emotional lability, but more severe cases may have negative affectivity accompanied by disinhibition (impulsivity) and dissociality (hostility). Such differences have probable implications for treatment planning and may help explain the inconsistent results of treatment RCTs in those with borderline personality disorder.

While the multiple trait model is heuristically appealing and has face validity, there is no evidence of its applicability and usefulness in individuals with personality disorders. Diagnostic issues need to be carefully thought about or we may reduce patients to simple, if different, rigid categories, leading to the stalemate we are now in. The domains are dimensions, not categorical diagnoses, and need to be treated as such. While this adds complexity, it provides a way to more specifically target treatments to the patient.

8.18 Benzodiazepine Dependence and Personality

Another good reason for assessing personality in ordinary psychiatric practice is the difficult choice of prescribing a benzodiazepine for anxiety. It is commonly known that benzodiazepines are prone to create dependence in vulnerable individuals. This was known in patients on high dosage (usually as part of drug abuse) early on in their clinical use, but it was not until the early 1980s that they were recognised to create dependence at low dosage, as is normally used to treat anxiety (Tyrer, 1980; Petursson and Lader, 1981; Tyrer et al., 1981). Because of this concern in most countries of the world recommendations were made to practitioners to only prescribe benzodiazepines in the short term and withdraw them as soon as possible to avoid dependence (British Medical Association and Royal Pharmaceutical Society of Great Britain, 2010, pp. 205–206).

What has not been appreciated fully is that pathological dependence only occurs in a minority of individuals, probably about 35% of the population. One of the most important factors determining whether an individual develops dependence after taking a benzodiazepine is their personality status. In a study published in 1983 a cohort of patients had been on benzodiazepines for many years were gradually withdrawn from their medication after all had been switched to diazepam, as this drug comes in many different dosage strengths.

In the study half the patients were randomised to early withdrawal and the other half to later withdrawal. The personality status of all patients was assessed with the Personality Assessment Schedule (PAS) at the beginning of the study. Forty-four per cent of the patients developed significant withdrawal symptoms and it was found that personality status was a major determinant of withdrawal symptoms, with labile and impulsive personality characteristics (found most commonly in emotional dysregulation) having the main effects (Tyrer et al., 1983) (see Figure 8.1).

Ever since this time PT has assessed personality status in every patient before considering treatment with benzodiazepines. Those who clearly have personality disturbance with negative affective and/or anankastic features have been warned that once they start

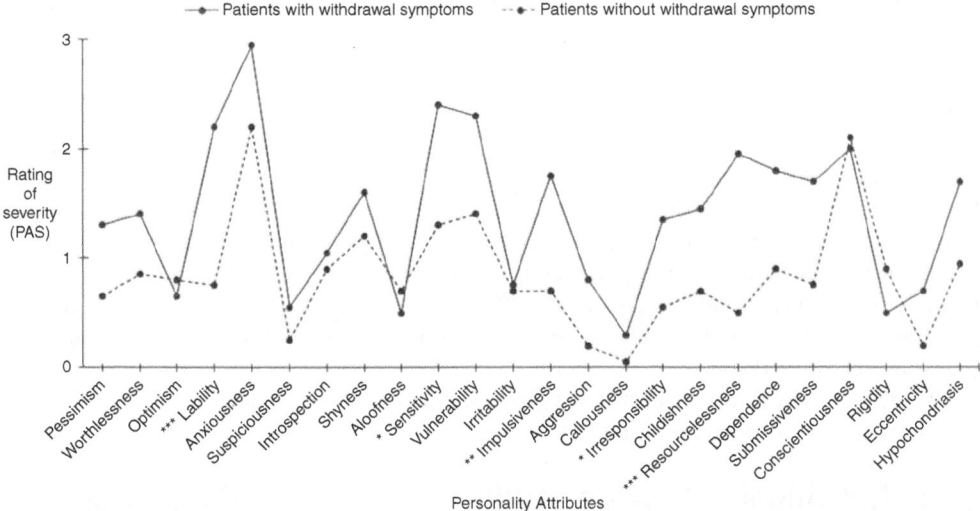

Figure 8.1 Personality characteristics (measured by the Personality Assessment Schedule (PAS)) measured in patients on long-term benzodiazepine treatment before withdrawal of medication over six weeks. Those with emotionally unstable (borderline) personality features were more likely to have withdrawal problems. (From Tyrer et al., 1983. Redrawn and reproduced by permission of the editors and publishers of the Lancet).

benzodiazepines they are unlikely to withdraw from them easily unless they take them in intermittent flexible dosage so that tolerance does not develop. A psychological treatment is then normally recommended as an alternative.

Exactly similar findings were found in a later study by Schweizer et al. (1998) in a study of 171 patients withdrawn from benzodiazepines in the USA. They concluded that a 'risk–benefit assessment' should be made 'in the planning of benzodiazepine treatment for patients with anxious symptomatology'.

So here we have clear evidence that knowledge of personality status should affect practice in the form of treatment. One of the reasons the relationship between personality and dependence has not become more widely known is that those prescribing benzodiazepines (mainly initiated in primary care) rarely consider any formal assessment of personality. We would argue that the wider use of ICD-11 will make an appropriate personality assessment more readily available so that the blanket refusal to prescribe a benzodiazepine that is so common in many areas can change to a more nuanced approach (Silberman et al., 2020).

8.19 Outcome of Personality Disorder

One of the reasons why personality disorder has attracted such connotations of stigma is the belief that fundamentally it is untreatable. The same stigma used to be attached to mental illness. The notion of a permanent scar created by a hot iron is a corrosive one. It implies that everyone can see the scar from the time it was created until death.

The only satisfactory way of determining outcome is by long-term prospective studies. Long-term in this context means many years, long beyond the 2–5 year span that many consider to be long term. Lesser ways of estimating the outcome include (a) examining trends in the age range of personality disorder, (b) individual follow-up studies from clinical populations and (c) extrapolating from trait population studies.

8.20 Trends in Age Range

When representative epidemiological studies of the population and of psychiatric subjects are examined there are several common features. Antisocial and histrionic personality features are more common in young people (many with so-called conduct disorder come into this group) but much less so in older ones (Tyrer, 1988; Cohen et al., 1994; Coid et al., 2006). Obsessional and schizoid personality disorders are more common in the elderly than in the young (Tyrer, 1988; Engels et al., 2003; Schuster et al., 2013). These data are not conclusive, not least as those with antisocial characteristics tend to die at a younger age (Krasnova et al., 2019).

But these findings do suggest that there are changes in personality disorder over time and that these conditions are not all the same.

8.21 Individual Follow-Up Studies from Clinical Populations

The best known of all long-term follow-up studies in psychiatric practice is the comprehensive one of Mary Zanarini and her colleagues at McLean Hospital and the University of Harvard. This study involved repeated assessments in 275 patients with borderline personality disorder at 4-yearly intervals over a 24-year period. This was not a typical population; all the patients at the time of recruitment were in-patients with borderline personality disorder, and over the course of follow-up there was a considerable amount of treatment, especially pharmacotherapy (Zanarini et al., 2003; Zanarini et al., 2012b; Zanarini et al., 2015; Zanarini et al., 2019).

The results were striking, as they appeared to show that borderline personality disorder had a very good long-term outcome. Remission rates (i.e. absence of disorder) were 20%, 50% and 85% after 1, 2 and 10 years, respectively. (These were so impressive that colleagues would joke that if you wanted to be treated successfully you should make a beeline for McLean Hospital.) But the findings were to some extent replicated by similar ones from the large Collaborative Longitudinal Personality Disorders study (Gunderson et al., 2011). In this study several other personality disorders were assessed as well as borderline and after 10 years 85% had remitted. At this time only 12% had relapsed. But the findings were not all positive. Social functioning is significantly impaired in those with personality disorder, more so than in major depression (Skodol et al., 2002). This impaired function is now taken into account with the Levels of Personality Function Scale in DSM-5, which shows strong agreement with general social function (Buer Christensen et al., 2020).

Borderline personality disorder was also found to show poorer social function than other personality disorders (Gunderson et al., 2011), suggesting that it would be unwise to trumpet remission rates alone when discussing outcome.

In the long-term, Nottingham Study of Neurotic Disorder patients with anxiety and depression were involved in a randomised trial of drug and psychological treatments and followed up for 30 years (Yang et al., 2021). Personality status was also assessed in the same form at baseline, 2 years, 12 years and 30 years by face-to-face interviews. The results showed that in this population most patients changed their personality status over the 30-year period. The greatest stability shown in those who had no personality disturbance at baseline, but overall there was change to greater pathology over follow-up than improvement, with many patients oscillating between improvement and deterioration (Yang et al., 2021) (Figure 8.2). In this study those with borderline pathology at baseline showed the least changes over 30 years, but there was an increase in those with schizoid, obsessional and dependent pathology. This is consistent with the results of three other longitudinal studies (Clark, 2005).

8.22 Extrapolation from Trait Population Studies

If personality disorder is truly on a spectrum, including those with less personality pathology, then one would expect a similar set of findings from trait population studies. It is first apposite to point out that when trait change is compared with personality disorder change traits are much more consistent (Hopwood et al., 2013). Generally, most people retain positive personality features as they mature from early adulthood to middle age. They become more dominant, agreeable, conscientious and emotionally stable (Caspi et al., 2005). The greatest consistency of personality traits is between the ages of 50 and 70 (Roberts and DelVecchio, 2000), but the study of changes in personality status after the age of 70 has been generally neglected. Studies of longevity show that is related to personality with those of greater emotional stability and conscientiousness leading to longer life,

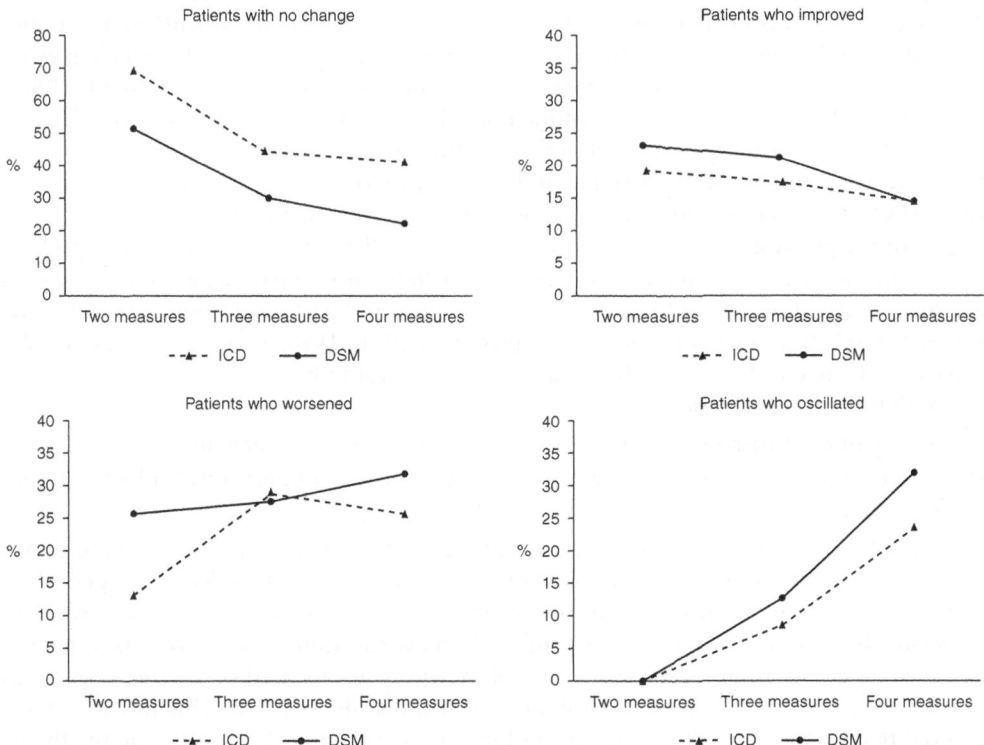

Figure 8.2 Illustration of degree and nature of change in personality status in anxious and depressed patients using ICD and DSM personality disorder groupings. These were tested on four occasions over a 30-year period. (Reproduced from Yang et al., 2021, by permission of the editor and publishers of Australian and New Zealand Journal of Psychiatry).

even though, as noted in Chapter 6, this can be interpreted in several ways. What is also clear is evidence of shorter lives in those with a greater measure of disagreeableness in the Big Five group, including due to cardiovascular disease among many others (Miller et al., 1996).

From these three sets of enquiries, it can be concluded that personality disorders, unlike personality traits, are very prone to change and the original notion that they were persistent and ingrained has to be abandoned. The changes over time are generally positive but for those who have personality disorder diagnosed in adult life the outcome is much less rosy. This seems to be particularly true for those with personality problems in the negative affective domain. The domains of detachment and anankastia also become more prominent in older age and frequently progress to frank personality disorder.

8.23 Conclusions

There is now much published about the treatment of personality disorders and the consensus, not always easy to achieve, has to be that psychological treatments have some efficacy and that pharmacological ones have very little or none. But when you delve further into the degree of efficacy, you come across uncomfortable truths. The delving is difficult, but once you get past the verbal palisades of psychological interpretation, theoretical models and relational continuity, there is little to show for intensive efforts to improve the lot of people with personality disorder. The trial evidence, after a generation of effort, is unimpressive. The largest effect sizes (the measure of superiority over a control treatment) in the studies that have had the biggest impact have been found with a total sample of 44 (Linehan et al., 1991), 38 (Bateman and Fonagy, 1999b), 90 (Clarkin et al., 2007) and 124 patients (Blum et al., 2008). By contrast, the results of the unequivocally negative findings of Schulz et al. (2008) comparing olanzapine and placebo, McMurran et al. (2017) in the PEPS study, and Crawford et al. (2018) of lamotrigine and placebo, recruited 319, 309 and 276 patients, respectively. Cristea et al. (2017) have carried out an excellent meta-analysis and systematic review of the psychotherapy trials and have concluded there are some benefits of psychotherapy in borderline personality disorder, but conclude with a warning message: 'the effects are small, inflated by risk of bias and publication bias, and particularly unstable at follow-up'. So the only trials that come up to the Johnson criterion (1998) are the negative ones. We leave it to the reader to decide which findings are the best to believe.

With this sparse evidence of value we have to ask ourselves two questions:

(a) Do any of the treatments for personality disorder have lasting benefits?
(b) Does the introduction of the ICD-11 classification offer an opportunity for better studies to evaluate efficacy?

We are not sure of the answer to the first and at present the jury is still out. It is an important question as in the absence of intervention many personality disorders may persist or worsen. But we are optimistic about the second question. The assessment and treatment of personality disorders using ICD-10 and DSM-5 classification models with its unhelpful categories has had limited success. Nearly all the effort has focused on the heterogeneous borderline groupings, with a little leaking out to the antisocial one. This has essentially showed that all structured therapies (including structured clinical care without any theoretical model) are moderately and equally effective for a limited time. Drug treatments have fared even worse, with inconsistent and conflicting recommendations, including non-recommendations of any drug. We have to conclude that there has been no real progress in the last 20 years (Newton-Howes and Mulder, 2020).

ICD-11 provides a new way of examining personality pathology. The diagnosis based on severity is the most relevant variable in deciding who to treat, how to treat and how to measure outcome. The trait domains, congruent with normally distributed personality traits, allow further formulation of the needs of individual patients. Our hope is that groups such as 'moderate personality disorder in the negative affectivity domain' (as well as many others) can be identified more clearly and allow treatment to be tailored to individual patients. It moves away from a simplistic focus on borderline symptoms and encourages more consideration of the wide range of personality pathology found in most patients. The ICD-11 model at least offers a way forward. While its success or not will only be apparent after a period of evaluation and data gathering, it provides an approach for assessment and treatment much closer to the evidence than the one we have left behind.

Moderating the Stigma
of Personality Disorder

This chapter addresses one of the most serious matters in the study of personality disorder that is in danger of permanently handicapping understanding and treatment. It could, in the end, sabotage research and keep the subject as an esoteric one where only a small number of zealots communicate among themselves. It is a concern that the two highly respected handbooks recently published on personality disorder (Livesley and Larstone, 2018; Lejuez and Gratz, 2020) have no chapters or discussion sections on the stigma of personality disorders, despite its importance.

Put simply, we have to address the following questions: If it is acceptable to use the word 'personality', why is it unacceptable to use the term 'personality disorder'? If we conclude that the stigma of personality disorder is significantly greater than the stigma attached to other mental disorders, what can we do to reduce or remove it?

9.1 Stigma in Psychiatry

Let us consider depression as an example. In the distant past, people were never quite sure whether this referred to a mood or an illness, and so the terms 'depressive illness' and, much later, 'major depressive disorder' were used to emphasise the illness component. By using the word 'illness' or 'disorder', we are already introducing an element of stigma, but not a massive one (even though some who decry the use of labelling seem to think so). In the 1930s and 1940s, the word 'depression' was generally avoided unless it was regarded as very severe, when it could be called melancholia. The notion of personality was already well established by that time and was regarded as a very acceptable component of enquiry in all psychiatric disorders, but it was seldom described as a disorder.

But when 'psychiatric disorders' did become respectable, at least temporarily (as since the publication of DSM-5, they are back in the pig trough), there was a lessening of stigma, but from the comments people made to Lewis Wolpert, himself a sufferer from depression who was not averse to disclosure, it was only partial (Wolpert, 2001):

> There can be no doubt that there is considerable stigma associated with depression. I am repeatedly congratulated for being so brave, even courageous, in talking so openly about my depression. I, in fact, am a 'performer' and there is no bravery, but these comments show how others view depression and that it is highly stigmatised. An example of how stigma can present a particularly difficult problem for sportsmen is provided by the case of a professional footballer, Stan Collymore who played for England. He had a severe depression and his career went into a rapid decline. He says that he can never forgive the Aston Villa manager for the way he reacted to his depression. He told him to pull his socks up and that his idea of depression was that of a woman living on a 20th floor flat with kids.
>
> (Wolpert, 2001, p. 222)

So it is clear that stigma is still alive and well in general psychiatry, but we should also acknowledge that public campaigns, and expositions by people of influence such as Norman Sartorius (Sartorius and Schulze, 2005), Graham Thornicroft (Thornicroft, 2006), Stephen Fry, Princess Diana and other members of the Royal Family, have helped to lessen it in recent years.

9.2 Stigma of Personality Disorder

The stigma of personality disorder is in a different league. It is not only the general public, people who receive the diagnosis, health professionals and physicians in general, who embrace stigma in their handling of personality disorder, but psychiatrists themselves are major culprits. First we need to understand why 'personality disorder' attracts so much opprobrium. Much of the criticism is samizdat criticism, 'under the radar' comments, but it is still widely expressed.

9.3 Health Professionals' Views of Personality Disorder

It is useful to look at the stigma of personality disorder from several perspectives. First, it is instructive to find out how commonly personality disorder is diagnosed in clinical practice, whether the proportions fit in with epidemiological data, and what the attitudes of health professionals are towards the condition.

If you compare these figures with actual diagnostic practice, you find a 10–20-fold difference; personality disorder is hardly ever diagnosed in out-patients, and very rarely in in-patients (3–4% internationally).

This mismatch is illustrated in Figures 9.1 and 9.2. On the basis of epidemiology, we would expect at least 60% of Finnish patients admitted to hospital would have a diagnosis of personality disorder. The proportion of actual diagnoses is 20-fold lower.

There could be several reasons for this. The epidemiologists could have got it all wrong. They may have misinterpreted the diagnostic descriptions. This is highly unlikely; assessors go through a strict review process and have no innate bias. They are attempting to be accurate. The diagnostic guidelines may themselves be too crude and over-inclusive, so more are diagnosed in surveys than the true figure. But this is not enough to explain a 20-fold difference. The other explanation is that clinicians at all levels are afraid to make the diagnosis of personality disorder even when it is staring at them in their faces, or they have a completely different view of personality disorder from that put forward by diagnostic guidelines.

Our colleague, Giles Newton-Howes, examined this in a study of diagnosis in community mental health teams. Forty per cent of the sample had a personality disorder assessed by the researchers (Newton-Howes et al., 2010), as might be expected from the data in Figure 9.1. But, as the clinicians also made assessments of personality disorder, Newton-Howes took this project a stage further. He wanted to compare four groups by personality status to see if there were important differences that could account for the differences in clinician or instrument-derived diagnosis. These groups were: (i) those without clinical or instrument-derived personality disorder; (ii) those without instrument-derived but with clinically derived personality disorder; (iii) those with personality disorder identified by instrument but not clinical diagnosis ('covert personality disorder'); and (iv) those with clinical diagnosis and instrumental diagnosis of personality disorder ('overt personality disorder'). Those with covert personality disorder constituted the majority (70.2%). Only

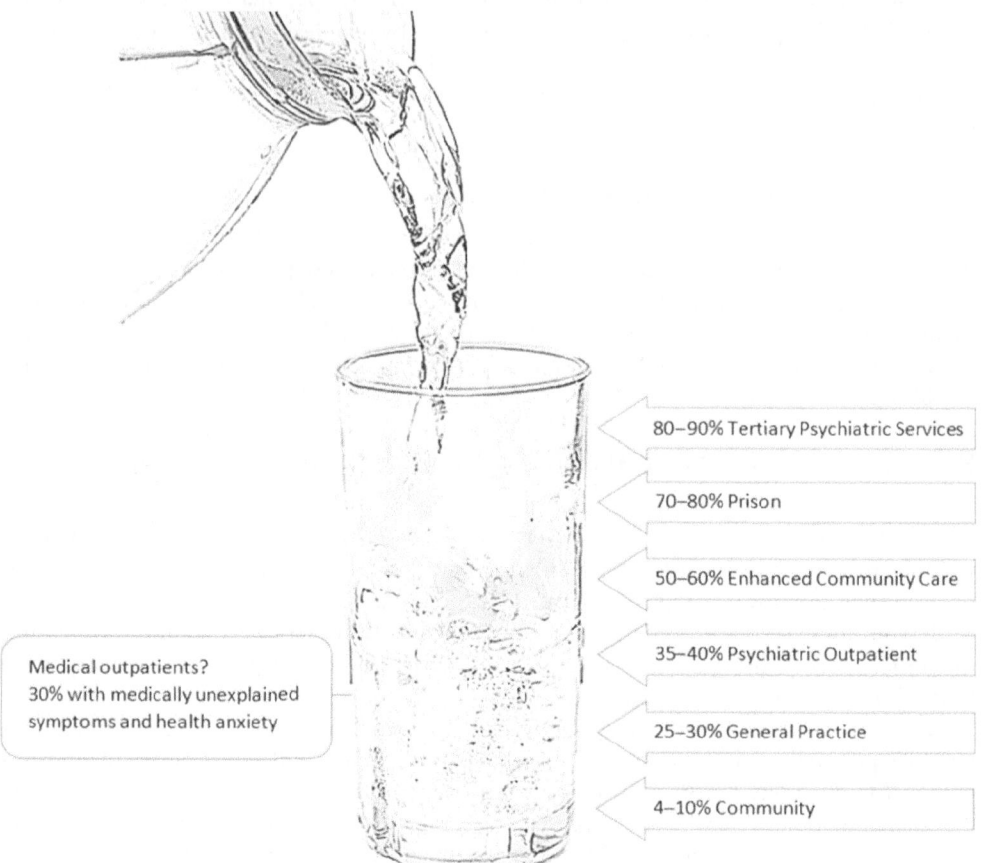

Figure 9.1 The epidemiological jug of personality disorder, showing the average proportions with these disorders in different settings.

three (2.7%) were diagnosed by the clinician as having personality disorder not shared by the research instrument.

The results were striking. There was no difference between the 'covert' and 'overt' groups in terms of their social functioning and symptomatology, but the ones diagnosed as personality disordered were wrongly perceived as more chaotic, difficult to engage and to be generally more disordered. Put simply, those labelled as having personality disorder were wrongly seen as more difficult to manage than the others only identified by the researchers.

So the conclusion made was unequivocal:

> An awareness of a personality disorder diagnosis is associated with a clinician belief that patients will be harder to manage. Objective measures of potential confounders do not explain why this group should be harder to manage. One explanation of this finding is that the label 'personality disorder' is stigmatizing. This may also explain the disparity between clinical and research assessments of personality disorder.
>
> (Newton-Howes et al., 2008b, p. 572)

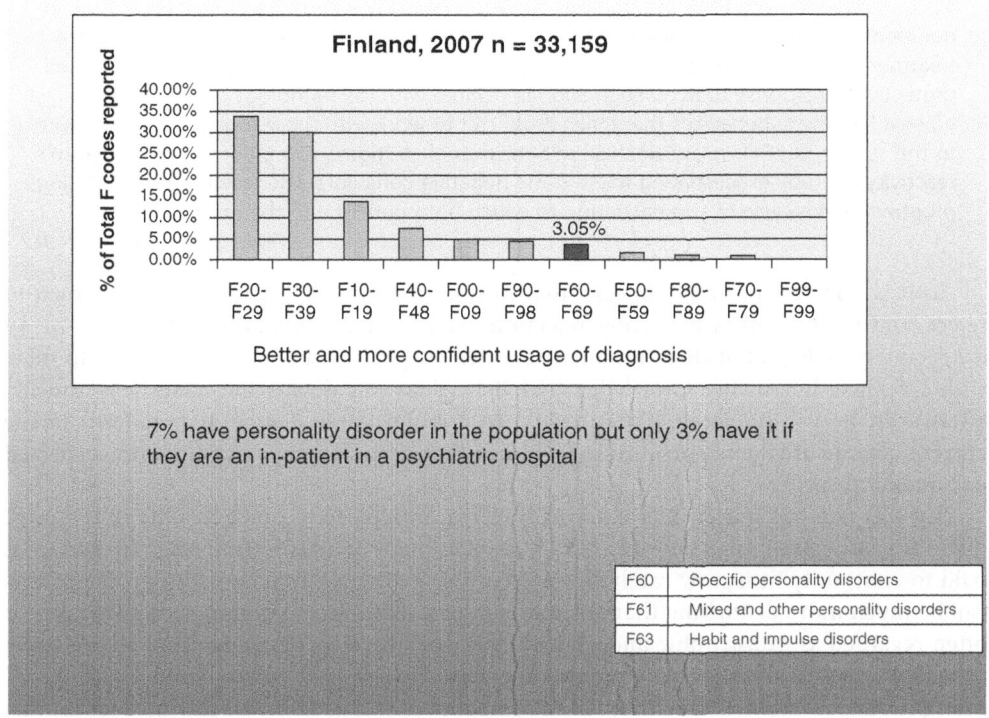

Figure 9.2 National statistics for ICD-10 diagnoses of patients admitted to Finnish psychiatric hospitals in 2007 (NB. ICD-10 code F60-69 = personality disorders). Note the mismatch with Figure 9.1.

9.4 Stigma Perceived by Patients

After reading the above, it is easy to see why patients should feel stigmatised by the diagnosis of personality disorder. A set of expectations has been set up in the clinician's mind best summarised by the Latin expression 'caveat emptor'. This is commonly translated as 'let the buyer beware', but when people with perceived personality disorder are seen it gets extended to 'this patient is going to be very difficult, so to save trouble, do not get too involved and get them off your hands as soon as possible'.

This is most commonly seen with the most commonly diagnosed personality disorder, borderline or emotionally unstable personality disorder, a diagnosis that we have argued earlier (see Chapter 4) offers little help to either patient or therapist and is ripe for confusing signals.

The stigma of misplaced expectation is described well by Aviram and colleagues (2006), especially with a population that is sensitive to rejection:

The stigma associated with borderline personality disorder (BPD) may affect how practitioners tolerate the actions, thoughts, and emotional reactions of these individuals (*i.e. those with likely borderline features* [our italics]). It may also lead to minimizing symptoms and overlooking strengths. In society, people tend to distance themselves from stigmatized populations, and there is evidence that some clinicians may emotionally distance themselves from individuals with BPD. This distancing may be especially problematic in treating patients with BPD; in addition to being unusually sensitive to rejection and abandonment, they may react negatively (e.g., by harming themselves or withdrawing from treatment) if they perceive such distancing and rejection. Clinicians' reactivity may be self-protective in response to actual behavior associated with the pathology. As a consequence, however, the very behaviors that make it difficult to work with these individuals contribute to the stigma of BPD. In a dialectical relationship, that stigma can influence the clinician's reactivity, thereby exacerbating those same negative behaviors. The result is a self-fulfilling prophecy and a cycle of stigmatization to which both patient and therapist contribute.

(Aviram et al., 2006, p. 249)

So it is a matter of great concern that in this situation the therapist is often keen to reject, and the patient is expecting rejection even though not wanting it. It may be an exaggerated analogy, but there are many species of spider where the male wishes to mate with a female, but in the knowledge that if he does not depart the scene very quickly afterwards, he will be eaten. This anxiety, to a much lesser degree, is paralleled in the current climate of stigma surrounding a junior therapist meeting a patient with suspected personality disorder.

But this nervous initial interaction is now commonplace in practice. One of the most disturbing aspects of modern psychiatry is discontinuity of care. Even though lip service is paid to continuity, it is now rarely followed and for those with personality problems this can be much more disturbing than for many others. The loss of contact with a therapist is often regarded as catastrophic and, in a stigmatised universe, it can so often be misinterpreted. Barbara Taylor, an ex-patient of Friern Hospital in North London, who had multiple difficulties, including those in the personality arena, describes the internal conflict of therapy loss very well in her book, *The Last Asylum: A Memoir of Madness in Our Times*:

Dr D won't see me any more when I go to the Day Hospital
    What? Not at all?
    No. Well, only in ward rounds. Like all the other patients.
    Like her other patients? You mean she has other patients?
    What? What do you mean by that?
    The way you talk about her, it sounds like you're her only patient.
    Don't say that! That's so stupid! I know perfectly well I'm just another patient.

(Taylor, 2015, p. 176)

But of course the personality disordered patient isn't just another patient. He or she has special needs and continuity in dealing with them is more important than with many others. Our paradoxical system rarely recognises this and offers 'packages of care' that break up any consistency that might have developed.

Stigma Perceived by Psychiatrists

The roots of personality disorder are in pejorative and misogynist labelling and no amount of 'destigmatising' can change that. It's time we dropped the whole idea – neither medicine nor the law would be any the poorer if we did so.

(House, 2019a)

Allan House takes this further in his book:

There are real problems with this way of thinking [about personality disorder]. First, and rather obviously, it leads to an emphasis on the individual as the source of their problems and therefore downplays the role of other people and circumstances ...

Second, the diagnosis is often experienced as a way of saying 'the problem is about who you are as a person' and it is widely used in a critical or dismissive way by professionals in health and social care. The person on the receiving end can easily be stigmatised and become (rightly) angry – that anger then being used as further evidence of what's wrong with them. Not surprisingly, lots of people given this diagnosis don't like it and don't like the effect it has on the way others treat them.

This isn't to say that people don't have recognisable and enduring characteristics. We all know somebody who is particularly obsessional, prickly, paranoid or prone to emotional outbursts. Sometimes these characteristics do indeed seem important in explaining self-harm. For example, impulsivity is a tendency to act on the spur of the moment, without much thought and without consideration of the consequences. This characteristic is quite commonly associated with self-harm, especially when it is coupled with negative ways of thinking ...

What isn't right is elevating these observations into diagnostic statements – putting people into categories as if somebody's personality is a mental disorder – which is indeed where personality disorder sits in the main diagnostic systems used worldwide.

(House, 2019b, pp. 49–51)

We quote this at some length for two reasons. First, this is not an atypical response from the psychiatric profession, but it is expressed in print, and this is less common. Many people express similar opinions, but, at least currently, do so only in blogs, books or commentaries that are not peer-reviewed. So most of them are expressed in an indirect form. Second, we know Allan well, from his early professional days in Southampton and later in Nottingham. He has the merit of consistency. When we first presented data on the high prevalence of personality disorder in psychiatric patients in 1984, he had the same negative opinion of personality disorder that he has now, except at that time he was more concerned that it might be a diagnosis given only to the dispossessed and those of lower social class status (there is no evidence that this is actually true). But we emphasise that by quoting him and his negative views of personality disorder, this should not be interpreted as too specific; he is not an outlier. There are dozens of other psychiatrists who feel the same way, and unfortunately many may be so turned off by the title of this book they will never read these pages.

If our opinion formers and teachers have a negative view of the diagnosis as stigmatic, we feel they are merely compounding stigma, not reducing it. The circular argument goes: people labelled ('label' is a highly emotive word in this context) as having personality disorder are stigmatised (by me, by my colleagues of all disciplines and the world in general), and therefore I will never use the term except to criticise those who do, which will accentuate the stigma. As Oscar Wilde might have said, 'the only thing that is worse than talking about personality disorder is not talking about it'. We cannot ignore something that is very common.

So if we take all the figures together, it appears that more than 95% of people with personality disorders are undiagnosed in practice. So we have a situation where epidemiologists find a universally high prevalence of a diagnosis that clinicians studiously avoid. But there is one group that differs, those that regularly appear in court. It is only in the legal profession that personality disorder appears to be popular. Over the years we have seen several instances of people being unequivocally diagnosed as having personality disorder in court proceedings, but when you look at their clinical notes the subject is never mentioned.

So in clinical practice we feel it is offensive to say that people have personality disorders, both offensive to the patient and also to the health professional for having the temerity to use it, but in court there is no such sensitivity. Here stigma about disclosure seems to have been forgotten entirely. The consequence is that the general public is fed a steady stream of articles in the popular press about juicy criminal cases in which personality disorder takes centre stage. Bowen (2016) carried out a content analysis of 552 articles in the popular UK press, between 2001 and 2012, that made reference to personality disorder: 42% of these articles established a link between personality disorder and homicide. There was only a very small reduction in the frequency of these articles in the more recent years.

We can therefore conclude that the main reason why the threshold for the diagnosis of personality disorder is very much higher for practitioners than researchers is a direct consequence of stigma.

It seems to us there are at least ten elements contributing to the stigmatic perception of personality disorder:

1. The diagnosis is not a proper diagnosis; it is a value judgement.
2. The term is so badly defined, it does not mean anything.
3. Because we can identify all the features of personality disorder in ourselves, to use the term about others is an affront to them and ourselves.
4. The diagnosis is not like a diagnosis of any other disorder; it is a diagnosis of the person and, as such, is indelible and offensive.
5. You only use the diagnosis of personality disorder if you dislike the person, and this reflects badly on you as the diagnostician.
6. There is no need for the diagnosis as the pathology it describes can be covered by other descriptions.
7. The diagnosis is a life sentence of despair.
8. The diagnosis is misogynistic and reflects male prejudice.
9. The diagnosis is outmoded and should be supplanted by other more positive ones, including trauma disorders.
10. The diagnosis indicates that the person concerned is untreatable and by using it you are abandoning hope for them.

1. The diagnosis of personality disorder is a value judgement.

Values have become steadily more important in mental health as the limitations of conventional yardsticks have been more fully appreciated. One of the definitions of such judgements is that they are an expedient evaluation based upon a small amount of limited information, and are often needed to make decisions.

Because most psychiatric disorders lack comprehensive information to secure their scientific validity, value judgements come into use. In the case of personality disorder, it can be argued that it is too weak a category to be more than a value judgement. But on the other hand, it has practical value, more so in some areas of personality dysfunction than others.

As Sisti, Young and Caplan put it:

Values can drive practical considerations about where and how to divide up constellations of already agreed upon symptoms.

Or they might operate at a more fundamental level and influence what is considered to be dysfunctional or disordered behaviour in the first place.

(Sisti et al., 2013, p. 2)

The second of these sentences is appropriate for personality disorder in general; the first has been more subject to value judgements that are more suspect. Sisti et al. go on to say:

For example, feminist philosophers have argued that political and gender-based values about 'proper' feminine behaviour have driven particular disorder categories such as histrionic and borderline personality disorders and premenstrual dysphoric disorder.

(Sisti et al., 2013, p. 2)

There is a strong element of male value judgements in the descriptions of both histrionic and borderline personality disorder – in one old histrionic personality scale 'spends a lot of money on clothes' was a scored item – and the combinations of dramatic display, attention seeking, inappropriate flirtatious and seductive behaviour and excessive need for approval, together with what was formerly described as 'emotional incontinence', all smell nastily of male prejudice. When there is a large imbalance in the distribution of any personality disorder, it is right to ask questions about their value.

The evidence that there is considerable disparity between the frequency of diagnosis of emotionally unstable personality disorder across countries, with 30% less use in lower income countries than higher ones (Faiad et al., 2018), also suggest value judgements are at work.

But as we argue in many places elsewhere in this book, the old categories are redundant and their life is coming to an end.

2. The term is so badly defined, it does not mean anything.

We have sympathy with this viewpoint but feel that the main culprit is not the core diagnosis but, yet again, the uncritical embrace of the categorical system of classification. When it was possible to write that a patients had five, six, seven or even ten different allegedly comorbid personality disorders, the classification was rightly held up to ridicule.

One of the main purposes of this book is to show the advantages of a different classification based on severity in which all the stigmatic labels have been removed apart from 'borderline', currently just clinging on by its hems (see Chapters 2 and 4). The adoption of a single spectrum of personality disturbance cannot be accused of having no meaning. Everybody is on the spectrum somewhere.

3. Because we can identify all the features of personality disorder in ourselves, to use the term about others is an affront to them and ourselves.

We have to accept that personality disorder does not have the same valence as other diagnoses. Valence in this context may not be the ideal word, as we are looking for a word that describes the intrinsic feel of a phenomenon. Positive valence indicates favourability; negative valence disgust or unhappiness. No mental disorder has universal positive valence, but with increasing awareness some are becoming so. Personality disorder is an exception. For most people who have significant personality disturbance, help is never asked for even if required. In a study of medical students, Gardiner and her colleagues (2010) found that 12% had a personality disorder but 87% were Type R personalities (i.e. treatment resisting in that they did not want any assistance in tackling it). Why not? This is probably because, for most of us, our personalities are ego-syntonic, a term introduced by Sigmund Freud (1925) to describe mental processes that are accepted as part of the individual rather than separate and therefore alien. This has been described well by Stephen Fry:

> One division of mental health conditions that the general population has picked up on is the apparent distinction between *mood* disorders and *personality* disorders. Those of us who, like me, have suffered from the effects of bipolar disorder like to congratulate ourselves on the purity and constancy at least of our personalities. The illness, we say to ourselves, is like the weather. It comes from outside of who we are. We might be made alarmingly enthusiastic, exuberant, grandiose and overconfident when in the grip of elevated moods, or grumpy, silent, morose and pessimistic when depression descends on us like a leaden cloud, but inside we are ourselves, all right and tight. *Personality* disorders, that is what the boogeyman suffers from, they are dark and dangerous territory. To be told one suffers from such threatens our sense of self and the very ownership of who we are.
>
> (Fry, 2018)

So to be accused, or even hinting, of having a personality disorder is easily perceived as a personal affront, and to contemplate treating it is seen as assaulting the citadel of self. This will only change when we feel more comfortable with the personality spectrum on which we all belong. It will be helped even more by evidence, such as the study described in Chapter 8 on health anxiety, which suggests having a personality disorder has advantages when it comes to treatment.

4. The diagnosis is not like a diagnosis of any other disorder; it is a diagnosis of the person and, as such, is indelible and offensive.

This is an extension of the previous concern. It has face validity, but is it true? It assumes that clinicians using the term are using it in a completely different way from other diagnoses. But we argue that they are not. If we say that someone has a personality disorder, we are making the case that they have a collection of symptoms and behaviour that together coalesce into our understanding of the essence of personality disorder. We are not saying it is indelible or permanent (and we know it is not from even a casual look at Chapter 8). We are only making the case to the person concerned that at this point in time, and at others in the past, the features that are being displayed are those of an understandable and well-described condition called personality disorder. Most importantly, we are not predicting the prognosis by making the diagnosis.

Those who say it is a diagnosis of the person can argue that personality disorder differs from depression, anxiety or psychotic disorders as it differs by making a judgement that the essential core of the person is disordered. Other conditions can be regarded as extraneous: they have happened for some reason but are not part of your core being. But is this a sound argument, even if for some people it could be perceived as true? People with intellectual disability have disability of intelligence. We can attempt to camouflage this by saying they are 'slow learners' but we cannot make the case that they are hidden Einsteins. There is stigma that still attaches, and the rather shameful acronym, PWID (people with intellectual disability) is now being used frequently, allegedly to reduce stigma, but in fact serving to promote it.

5.   You only use the diagnosis of personality disorder if you dislike the person, and this reflects badly on you as the diagnostician.

This argument has some merit. It is very easy for a psychiatrist to conclude after a long day that an angry exchange with a patient can easily be interpreted as an interview with a 'typical borderline', when the exchange might be interpreted equally well as one illustrating a rude and irritable psychiatrist failing to listen to a patient. But this is a criticism more of the diagnosis than the diagnoser. If you still retain a diagnosis where a single negative interaction permits the entry of a diagnosis, it will be allowed expression. Thus, as we have mentioned earlier in Chapter 4, the continuing professional belief, 'personality disorder, the patients psychiatrists dislike' (Lewis and Appleby, 1988), unchanged after 30 years (Chartonas et al., 2017), becomes ingrained in continued stigma.

The old categorical labels have enhanced the stigma of personality disorder several-fold, and have not been helped by Donald Trump's critics, who toss them around like confetti. The categories of disorder such as narcissistic, histrionic and schizotypal have become a laughing stock, hardly ever used in practice but wheeled out to beat politicians and those we oppose mercilessly, so adding to stigma. This has infected the psychiatric community also. The only clinicians concentrating their attention on people with personality disorder are forensic psychiatrists, who have no choice, since all their patients have personality disorder, and specialists in the borderline group, who have invested greatly in the subject and cannot tolerate it being abandoned. All health professionals avoid using the term in their normal practice, except, interestingly, when they perceive the patient concerned is difficult to manage, even though comparison with others not so diagnosed shows they have the same degree of dysfunction and symptomatology (Newton-Howes et al., 2008b).

As a consequence of the poor way in which we, and here the collective 'we' includes all in health practice, have described, classified and labelled personality disorder so woefully, there have been powerful moves to get rid of the term altogether:

> This diagnostic label should be helpful because it can act as a gateway for individuals to access the care they need. Unfortunately all too often it can be used as a reason to reject individuals from services. Most of us would rather not use the term at all. In writing this document, it has been hardest of all for us to get consensus on what words we should use to talk about the problems and difficulties people with this diagnostic label experience. We would like to abandon the term 'personality disorder' entirely. The label is controversial for good reasons: it is misleading, stigmatizing and masks the nature of the problem it is supposed to address, adding to the challenges which people experience.
>
> (MIND, 2018)

This is not an outlandish statement by a fringe group of discontents. It was published by MIND with contributions from experts across the field of psychiatry and psychology and supported by the British Psychological Society (BPS), Royal College of Nursing, Royal College of General Practitioners, Centre for Mental Health, Anna Freud Centre and a mental health trust (Barnet, Enfield and Haringey). Norman Lamb, a former MP and Minster of Health, was also a key figure in creating the document.

The BPS was the most vocal of the organisations behind the document. But this gives greater credence to the Society than is justified. A group within the Society created the Power Threat Meaning Framework (PTMF), which was never authorised as a policy for the BPS, even though that is often implied. It consists of a group of senior psychologists (seven) and high profile service campaigners (two) who spent five years developing the PTMF as an alternative to more traditional models based on psychiatric diagnosis. Personality disorders are only one of conditions in their sights but has been most prominent recently.

Lucy Johnstone, one of the founders of PTMF summarises the framework in these words:

> The Power Threat Meaning Framework can be used as a way of helping people to create more hopeful narratives or stories about their lives and the difficulties they have faced or are still facing, instead of seeing themselves as blameworthy, weak, deficient or 'mentally ill'.
> (British Psychological Society)

Note that the focus here is not on helping people to relieve distress or suffering but somehow to reframe their problems as stories. Sorry, most people with problems with their mental state do not want stories. Some may, but all should have a choice, and PTMF does not brook any alternatives. The 'research' presented in support of the PTMF is non-existent, merely opinion pieces from authors challenging standard orthodoxies. The Framework comes from *Alice in Wonderland*, a pretty good story, with the Mad Hatter representing power, the Red Queen as threat, leaving it to the Walrus and the Carpenter to provide the meaning.

So the PTMF does not represent mainstream psychological opinion; it is the product of a lobby group, not a serious scientific contender. It has been dismissed by others in the BPS of much greater standing:

> The idea that a small group of psychologists aligned with a couple of closely aligned experts by experience can produce a framework (which was not peer reviewed nor subject to any primary research) that would then be implemented nationally is patently absurd.
> (Salkovskis, 2019, lecture at Royal College of Psychiatrists)

There are relevant aspects of the PTMF criticism that still need addressing in personality disorder – it is not complete nonsense – and these are discussed in the Chapter 10. But do not let these seduce you into thinking that this head-on challenge is a way forward for mental health. There are several models of mental disorder that co-exist reasonably well together and these can be integrated (Tyrer, 2013). The mistake is to line them up as warring parties.

Alternative models of care and diagnosis come about when existing ones are failing. There is no doubt that the services available for personality disorder are less than adequate, but this is no reason to conclude that the blame can be dumped almost entirely on the term 'personality disorder', and for this to be eliminated. Half of the population will die of cancer and most are under the care of services when they die, but this is not a reason to campaign for the abolition of 'cancer' as a stigmatising negative diagnosis, even though in the past it was regarded as such.

The solution to the problem, as we have been illustrating throughout this book, is to provide better evidence. Throughout the MIND document there are solutions offered, some of which might be a great step forward, but they are untested. In a commentary on the consensus statement Steve Chaplin of the journal *Progress in Neurology and Psychiatry*, looking for such a solution, wrote:

> The statement calls for a new approach to care for people with personality disorder. Currently, they are not well served by the ways in which psychological care or medication are traditionally delivered because many have such complicated problems that mental health services alone do not provide the help they need. There is evidence that a primary care-based service delivering psychological therapies and support for GPs for people with complex needs can improve outcomes compared with the Improving Access to Psychological Therapies programme and also reduces demand on GPs and emergency and outpatient departments.
>
> (Chaplin, 2018)

Chaplin was probably right. The Primary Care Psychotherapy Consultation Service (PCPCS) was set up in London by the local NHS Trust (Tavistock and Portman) to help GPs in their own surgeries and to help primary care staff deal with chronic problems. The people referred were mainly those with chronic mood and personality disorders, including many with medically unexplained symptoms. Although no control group was included, the savings on consultations was impressive in all groups (Parsonage et al., 2014). We have other evidence that liaison of primary care psychiatry with mental health practitioners going into surgeries regularly is a very effective use of resources and reduced admissions (Tyrer et al., 1989; Williams and Balestrieri, 1989; Tyrer et al., 1990). This approach is worth testing more fully in those with personality disorder and medically unexplained symptoms, especially now we have evidence that those with personality disorder are preferentially helped.

There are some people who scorn the diagnosis of personality disorder because it exemplifies psychiatric positivism. Such as approach is 'earnestly committed to discerning what is *wrong* with people before "treating" them' (Pilgrim, 2018). We hope that we have convinced you already that personality assessment is indeed a useful precursor to treatment, but if not, please read the rest of this even more carefully.

6. There is no need for the diagnosis as the pathology it describes can be covered by other descriptions.

This criticism also has some merit but is not a reason for avoiding the diagnosis. This argument goes along the lines of 'as personality is multifactorial, so are the disorders associated with it, and they cannot be combined together in a single term, and any attempt to do so will always fail'. But is this not true of all diagnoses, and why the formulation of a problem is considered so important in a psychiatric history (see Chapter 1)? A classification term is convenient shorthand for communication, not a precise description. The term 'personality disorder', if used properly, indicates to another practitioner 'this patient currently has problems in relationships with others and this is creating problems in personal/social/occupational life that you need to take into account in assessment'. The domains in which the problems are manifest can be added, and the completed diagnosis gives a fairly comprehensive picture.

7. The diagnosis is a life sentence of despair.

This criticism can be expressed in greater detail from the immediate perspective of a patient on receiving the diagnosis: 'You are telling me that all my problems are linked to my personality and, by saying it is disordered, you are condemning me to the deprivation of valuable treatments and the assumption that I will never improve, no matter how hard I try.'

All the clauses in this statement can be challenged. Personality disorder is not an all-encompassing diagnosis and is known to be associated with many other mental disorders. Each of these can be treated, but we argue that if the presence of personality disorder is acknowledged also then better management will ensue. The presence of personality disorder should not mean that effective treatments for other disorders are denied, even though in practice they still are (Williams et al., 2020). This is a criticism of the prescribers, not the diagnosis. There is also abundant evidence that personality can change for the better, irrespective of any treatment that might be offered, so the canard that improvement is impossible can be dismissed unequivocally.

8. The diagnosis is misogynistic and reflects male prejudice.

This is one of the more ludicrous criticisms. Some personality disorders are more common in men than women (Eaton & Greene, 2018). Personality disorder is extremely common in men, more so than anxiety, depression and other common mental illnesses. We do not claim that a male psychiatrist diagnosing an anxiety disorder in a female patient is misogynistic, so why pile the offending adjective on to the psychiatrist who uses the term personality disorder? Histrionic personality disorder is definitely misogynistic, so few will cry about its loss.

9. The diagnosis is outmoded and should be supplanted by other more positive ones, including trauma disorders.

Every diagnosis in psychiatry has been shown to be more common in those that are abused or suffer trauma at an early age than those who are not so exposed. If the trauma is a major factor in the condition, then it is appropriate to use the diagnosis of post-traumatic stress disorder (PTSD). In the ICD-11 classification it is also possible to make the diagnosis of Complex PTSD if the time line between the exhibition of the trauma and manifestations of disorder is a more convoluted one. But, despite this association, most people with any disorder, including personality disorders, have not suffered significant trauma. You cannot airbrush the evidence away, even though it is possible to argue that before the expansion of diagnosis to include Complex PTSD some may have been inappropriately diagnosed as personality disordered. Trauma is often a relevant factor in diagnosis but is never the whole story (see Chapter 4).

10. The diagnosis indicates that the person concerned is untreatable and by using it you are abandoning hope for them.

This may have been true in the past but is certainly not now. Almost every chapter in this book indicates the presence of effective treatment. We agree that some clinicians still hold to this view but they are steadily diminishing in number.

9.5 Solution to the Stigma of Personality Disorder

It is unarguably the case that personality disorder is associated with more stigma than other mental disorders, and personality disordered patients get more than their fair share. So how do we remove or reduce it? The standard response is to change the name, as we have done repeatedly with mental handicap over the years.

Our solution is to stress the fact that everybody is on the same spectrum of personality disturbance; it might be viewed as more than one spectrum but for diagnostic purposes there is only one. Some can be placed on the left on the non-disordered end, and others, at least at a certain point in time, can be placed on the right. By explaining to people currently diagnosed as personality disorder, 'you are somewhere to the right of this scale, but you have the potential to move to the left', the stigma of diagnosis is greatly reduced. It might even be expressed in percentage terms, so a patient can be told: 'You were at 75% last year but now you're at 65%.' It is still necessary, for medicolegal, technical and procedural reasons, to keep the term, personality disorder, but it need not be used until necessary for these other reasons.

To help in this task we have designated 25th May as International Personality Spectra Day and hope to host events around the world to impress on others that we are in a new world, where the stigma of personality disorder can no longer exist as we all have a little of it in our constitutions. But, in one way or another, we have to rid ourselves of the ridiculous notion that personality variation is acceptable except when it strays into disorder, when it becomes taboo. Health and illness are on a similar spectrum, and we are prepared to embrace the whole range; for personality disorders too we should be *omnia paratus*.

Chapter 10

What Needs to Be Done Now

If there is a volcano at Lisbon it cannot be elsewhere. It is impossible that things should be other than they are; for everything is right.

Pangloss, in Voltaire's Candide

In this last chapter we are offering an optimistic way forward, which if followed by all, will lead to wider use of the concept of personality disorder, better clinical care and greater understanding. This is not empty Panglossian optimism. Here we are not over-simplifying the challenges of personality disorder but showing that it can be taken out of the shadows of rejection and criticism and given its proper place in psychiatric practice and in general dialogue. We have failed both in the past, when we had prejudiced and negative views about all aspects of the subject, and also in the present, despite making some progress, by having an impractical and unnecessarily complicated classification system, and by over-selling a limited range of goods. These errors, far from opening up the subject, have led to over-specialisation and esoteric arguments that have left other health professionals out in the cold. Yet it is these health professionals, and also those involved in any form of care, seeing people with personality problems every day in their lives, whom we need to educate and encourage.

10.1 Dispose of Worn-Out Labels

We hope to have convinced you already that the categorical labels of the past are no longer of value, if indeed they ever were. The psychiatric profession has already discarded all the categories apart from antisocial (psychopathic/sociopathic) and borderline by simply never using them. Antisocial and borderline will survive for longer, not because they have greater justification, but because dropping them will feel to some as the same loss of control as falling off a cliff. These labels appear to offer a framework, a mechanism of understanding. But this is illusory, as these labels are heterogeneous. Here is one example of a condition thought up in the highest echelons of government, where much attention is given to personality disorder. Several years ago one of us (PT) was involved in a team assessment of a new diagnosis generated in 1999, 'dangerous and severe personality disorders' (DSPD) (Tyrer et al., 2007). The diagnosis was determined using Hare's Psychopathy Check List, revised (PCL-R) or International Personality Disorder Examination (IPDE). The requirements to be eligible for a treatment programme that nobody had evaluated were: The level of personality disorder required to be present to meet the definitional criteria:

a) PCL-R (Screening version) of 30 or more

   OR

b) PCL-R (Screening version) of between 25 and 29 *and at least* one personality disorder diagnosis using DSM-IV or ICD-10 other than anti-social personality disorder

OR

c) Two personality disorder diagnoses, one of which is anti-social personality disorder (or equivalent, using DSM-IV or ICD-10)(using IPDE) (Loranger et al., 1994; Loranger, 1999).

This looks on the surface to be good sensible science, using well-established measures. But just imagine an equivalent study of people with 'dangerous and severe hypertension'. The measurements would likely include measures of blood pressure over a period of time, other tests related to the effects of high blood pressure (e.g. renal and cardiac function) and possible ultrasound and other scans. All of these would be clearly related to hypertension.

If the requirements were changed to (a) a single measure of very high blood pressure, or (b) a lower blood pressure measurement together with at least one episode of headache, or (c) at least two episodes of symptoms that can occur in hypertension (headaches, blurred vision, chest pain, swelling of legs, nosebleeds), we would not be impressed by the accuracy of this new form of identification. Yet in the DSPD study this either/or assessment could determine the long-term future and the period of detention (often over 10 years) of the prisoners concerned.

In our study we found almost equal numbers of people with antisocial and borderline personality disorders in the patients we assessed, together with significant numbers of paranoid, obsessive–compulsive, narcissistic, schizoid and schizotypal personality disorders using the recommended instrument (IPDE; Loranger et al., 1994). We also found that one-third of the 75 prisoners we assessed did not have diffuse (now termed moderate in ICD-11) or severe personality disorders (Tyrer et al., 2009), mainly because the PCL-R scores were often very old and not reflecting current pathology.

What better illustration is there of a failed diagnostic system? Even the favoured categories performed poorly and the main differences between the groups were significantly greater scores on anxiety and depressive scales in those with borderline personality disorder than in others (Tyrer et al., 2007).

10.2 Embrace the Personality Spectrum

The ICD-11 classification, after initial doubts (Bateman, 2011; Gunderson and Zanarini, 2011), has been broadly welcomed. In particular, the arguments in favour of a dimensional or spectrum classification have been put strongly and cogently (Widiger and Oltmanns, 2016; Hopwood et al., 2018). The main criticisms made by Herpertz and her colleagues (Herpertz et al., 2017) were that:

i) There was no description of a well-functioning personality

ii) The new system of classification had not been tested adequately

iii) Suffering as opposed to functioning was not in the definitions

iv) The trait domains would ultimately decide clinical management

v) 'Relationship dynamics' were ignored, and

vi) Clinicians in the field much preferred prototype models of personality disorder.

These are not powerful arguments. No classification system defines those who are well – it is not an appropriate task. Any new classification is bound to be short of data at first; suffering, although important, is also not useful as a differentiating term and is rarely used in classification, and the last two criticisms refer specifically to borderline personality disorder. When jobbing psychiatrists, as opposed to experts who are naturally better disposed towards systems they know and have studied all their professional lives, hear about the ICD-11 classification their views are almost universally favourable as they see it as a way of escaping the log-jam of categories that block understanding.

Throughout this book we have been keen to give evidence for the statements we have made. It is also important to stress the mantra that 'absence of evidence is not evidence of absence'. Many of the disputed claims about personality disorder may well be true, but if there are no facts to support them, or if they are unverifiable through being statements of opinion only, they should not be repeated.

So when reading anything about personality disorder, whether in the popular press, social media or learned journals, you need to ask yourself the following questions:

a) What is the basis for this statement?
b) Can the basis be relied upon?
c) Has the author any pre-conceived views, and have they influenced the statement made?
d) Has the author any direct experience of the subject?

You could add that these questions should apply to any scientific commentary, but the reason why we stress them with personality disorder is that so much of the discourse on the subject is based on ignorance, prejudice or misguided attitudes. This is partly because personality disorder is not like any other medical or psychiatric disorder and does not follow established rules of description, concept or intervention. It is an orphan in a family world, overlapping but not belonging.

The key problem that differentiates the diagnosis of personality disorder from other mental disorders is that is not seen as an external affliction but as a statement about the person. You do not have a personality disorder: you are the disorder. But all the evidence in this book, especially the studies of outcome, show that this is a lie. Basic personality is you; personality disorder is not.

10.3 Integrate Borderline into the New Classification

It will not be as easy to get rid of 'borderline'. There is almost a mythology surrounding the term and myths are often more difficult to combat than mistaken scientific beliefs. Clearly those who are currently involved in research on borderline pathology will want to pursue their efforts to a sensible conclusion and the introduction of a new descriptive system will not prevent this.

But new research and planning of services will need to change. At present the many services for personality disorder across the world are misnomers; they are services for borderline only. Because there has been no classification of severity of personality disorder in the past, almost all treatment strategies have been focused on clinically diagnosed personality disorder, and we suspect, but cannot be sure, that most of the patients considered for treatment are in the moderate personality disorder group, with a few more serious examples in the severe category. These services will have to become more flexible. It is no longer good enough to only have a dialectical, cognitive analytical or mentalisation model available. The services offered are likely to be very different for people with pathology in the dissocial/negative affective domains from those in the negative affective/disinhibited and dissocial/detached ones, and also for those who have less severe pathology. These services in the past have all been focused on (severe) borderline pathology and have ignored the rest.

The ICD-11 classification also gives opportunity for new research. Comparison can be made between the alternative domain option of the 'borderline pattern' and the existing ones in ICD-11. This would be a good test of the diagnostic nomenclature and could lead (it probably will) to a separate grading of domain severity. This could show if the current borderline heterogeneous grouping can be usefully dissected into more homogeneous groups (Tyrer and Mulder, 2018).

There is a great deal of psychodynamic tradition invested in borderline. Bob Spitzer has admitted in the past to PT and to others, that at least part of his motivation for establishing a separate axis for personality disorders in DSM-III was the need to have support from psychodynamic colleagues for the new categorical system. 'There you are', he was able to say to these grumpy and disaffected colleagues who deplored the atheoretical stance of DSM-III, 'here you can have a whole axis of the classification for yourselves, and if you want to make it into a psychoanalytical zone of exclusivity you are quite at liberty to do so'. So many have embraced this enthusiastically. The multitudinous pathology of emotional deregulation leading to interpersonal conflict and despair allows for many interpretations and critics are quite right in saying that these cannot be covered by a single classification system.

But this can still be done within the bounds of the ICD-11 system. Ferment and torment can be separated into levels of severity even within a psychoanalytical framework. The ICD-11 system gives a real opportunity for borderline to be reassembled into groups that have consistent meaning. This will enable focused intervention instead of the current blunderbuss strategies linked to all-embracing rigid models.

10.4 For Health Professionals to Make an ICD-11 Diagnosis of Personality Status in Every Patient

This is perhaps the most difficult recommendation to implement. The initial reaction to what we are advising is that it is so ludicrous it can be dismissed out of hand. You cannot expect people who have no training in mental illness to be able to conclude when someone has personality problems. Sorry, think again; you can, because picking up the essentials of interpersonal dysfunction and other problems in relating to others is not difficult. Look how many people with no medical, or even any form of scientific qualification, have pronounced on the personality of Donald J. Trump.

We have presented evidence earlier that those with personality disorders consult with health professionals of all sorts much more frequently than other people. We do not have accurate figures, but it seems likely that 40% of attendees at surgical, medical and other hospital clinics have personality problems that are very likely to influence treatment. So our recommendation is that every hospital doctor and general practitioner should make an assessment of personality in *every* patient they see.

This need not be an attempt at a full diagnostic assessment. We suspect that many do pick up prominent personality features almost subliminally and alters their behaviour. One of us (PT) worked in an orthopaedic post early in his career. He was looking after two patients with slipped discs, both women in their mid-fifties, placed in adjacent beds. The same surgeon was responsible for both patients. But they were being treated differently. One was booked for an extensive laminectomy while the other was just being treated with bed-rest. The two patients chatted to each other and to me about the differences in their management. So PT decided to ask the surgeon why: 'Because one of them is a tiger and the other is a lamb', he replied. He did not realise that he was using a personality assessment to make a surgical decision. Many others probably act in the same way but it would be much better if this understanding was integrated into training.

10.5 Extend Research and Practice into Studies of Personality Disturbance at All Ages

There is a concern, partly understandable, that many children who show personality disturbance in adolescence in particular improve over time and do not manifest personality disorder in adult life.

But, as been stressed elsewhere in this book, we need to regard the diagnosis of disorder as one at a point in time. This is merely a statement that, at the present time in this person, personality function is abnormal. This can occur at any time from childhood onwards; it is not necessarily going to last. 'Emerging personality disorder', 'nascent personality disorder' and 'personality disorder in development' were all suggested during the meetings of our ICD-11 working group, but these failed to acknowledge that the manifestations of disturbance were essentially the same as that of the disorder later in life. They are all prevaricating terms that avoid uttering 'personality disorder' simply and baldly. While at present, the stigma of the term is still strong in many quarters, we have to acknowledge the studies that have demonstrated the relief that many patients, their relatives and practitioners show when their suffering has been acknowledged by a formal diagnosis delivered in a sympathetic and informed way (Ring and Lawn, 2019; Lester et al., 2020). This last point is critical; if the diagnosis is given positively, it becomes an explanation for all the uncertainty that has gone before.

So, for this reason our ICD-11 group decided eventually to allow for the diagnosis of personality disorder to be made at any age, with no upper or lower limits. This might be expected to increase the prevalence of personality disorder and in a preliminary study of three populations totalling 772 psychiatric patients (a combination of in-patients and out-patients), the prevalence did indeed increase by 7% (33.8% with ICD-10 and 40.4%) with ICD-11 (Tyrer et al., 2014b). But this is not a large increase. There is now gradual acceptance in child and adolescent psychiatry that personality disorder can be diagnosed in this population, but it needs to go further. This acknowledgement has been made for borderline personality disorder by Andrew Chanen and his colleagues in Australia, where for many years there has been a psychiatric service for this group, with considerable research interest (Chanen et al., 2008; Kaess et al., 2014).

Diagnosing personality disturbance is of particular relevance in adolescent self-harm, where in the past practitioners have tried desperately to avoid making the diagnosis of borderline or other personality disorders when even sufferers and their relatives recognise it for what it is, yet the name is never said. As borderline is such a fluid diagnosis infiltrating many parts of pathology, some prefer to use 'emotional dysregulation' instead of personality disorder. This is not unreasonable but, on its own, this term just describes the symptoms, not the rest of the personality disturbance and its implications.

None of these data indicate that personality disorder in childhood can be simply equated with that in adult life. Much is going on in childhood before personality status is fully formed. The differences in the developmental trajectories of personality have been well explored by De Clercq and her colleagues (Widiger et al., 2009; De Fruyt and De Clercq, 2014), and these do not exactly map on to adult personality dysfunction.

We also need to acknowledge the data that shows adolescent personality disorder, even though it may persist, has a much better outcome than adult diagnosed personality disorder (Skodol et al., 2007). Personality disorder in adolescence is not necessarily pervasive or permanent, and this is one of the very good reasons for intervening early in its management.

At the other end of life we remain remarkably ignorant about late onset personality disorder. Recent reviews of the subject (Mordekar and Spence, 2008; Bangash, 2020) illustrate the lack of knowledge on its prevalence and course, although all practitioners in old age psychiatry are aware of its importance. Such evidence that there is suggests that obsessional (anankastia) and schizoid (detached) characteristics become more pronounced in older people and antisocial (dissocial) ones become less so (Seivewright et al., 2002; Yang et al., 2021), but there are exceptions. Black, Baumgard and Bell (1995) found at follow-up that 42% of those with antisocial personality disorder had not improved. There is also evidence that major trauma later in life can also lead to long-term personality disturbance (Munjiza et al., 2019). Not surprisingly, borderline personality disorder has the most variable long-term outcome (Stone, 2016), but all personality groups can vary greatly and show evidence of plasticity over the long term (Newton-Howes et al., 2015a).

Because of this variation and tendency to change, the ICD-11 work group included late onset personality disorder in its description, but not in a formal sense. If a patient shows evidence of personality disorder after the age of 65 and if the manifestations have been present for at least two years, then the diagnosis of late-onset personality disorder can be made.

10.6 Improve Treatment Strategies across the Range of Personality Disturbance Using Many Providers

One of the main criticisms made by treatment-seeking people is that what is available for them is very limited. The panoply of treatments looks impressive, but they all have to be given by experts in the subject, of whom there are few, the duration of treatment seems to be rigid and far too long, and the waiting times seem interminable when you feel desperate for help. As a consequence of the gap in provision, there is both anger and optimism. The anger is often directed at the professionals who seem to control the entry to services, but the optimism comes from self-generated initiatives in community practice that are being tackled with increased confidence.

> We also share the view, held by many in our community practice, that biomedically-based pathology-focused assumptions remove powerful personal stories of oppression and abuse. These assumptions have the power to position specialist based services as the truly helpful ones and to de-emphasise the importance of services that work more holistically, less 'expertly' and often with a more widely socially focused agenda.
>
> (Ramsden et al., 2020)

When we consider the epidemiology of personality disorder, with one in ten of the population showing significant features, it is easy to understand this annoyance with specialist services that can only treat very few people, and then only for a period fixed in advance. Saying 'no' to all the others is not enough. But personality disorder is not a biomedical diagnosis, and all treatments are in the fray as we have very little to trumpet at present. Almost all the effective treatments we have for personality disorder are biosocial and environmental, and giving the diagnosis the boundaries of a classification helps to focus attention on problems that require specific interventions. Too much of the criticism is linked to the diagnostic name 'personality disorder', so often put in quotation marks as it seems dangerous to touch. But as that master diagnostician, Robert Kendell, put it:

> All our diagnostic terms are simply concepts, and the only fundamental question we can ask about them is whether they are useful concepts, and useful to whom?
>
> (Kendell, 1991)

If we remove borderline personality disorder from the discussion as a heterogeneous outlier, the evidence suggests the generic diagnosis of personality disorder is useful in law, in medicine and in psychiatric practice. It may not be particularly useful for a counsellor in private practice as the more serious levels of personality disturbance are seldom going to be experienced, but even in this group, there is some value in denoting the personality disturbance even if we are too nervous to acknowledge it.

Once one removes the etymological eight syllables of the diagnosis, the essence of many of these criticisms is 'There is too little treatment; it is reserved for only those severe enough to pass through the many hoops protecting specialised services, and we have to fill this gap somehow.' A fair comment. So the gaps have been partly filled, and when you have supportive long-term structures, like co-production of providers with patients, that go far beyond existing health technology protocols with long waiting times and fixed treatment sessions, they are embraced with enthusiasm. But we need more evidence of how these work, what outcomes we desire and whether there are any adverse effects or complications (McMurran, 2020). The advantage of the ICD-11 classification is that it acknowledges formally the high numbers of people with mild and moderate personality disorder. We are confident that new treatment approaches suitable for formal evaluation can be introduced for these.

There is now much energy, enthusiasm and commitment in the many enterprises being set up all over the world to help people with what are increasingly called 'complex emotional needs' rather than personality disorder. When Benefield and Haigh (2020) write 'we need to focus on the common experience we all have of a birth-to-death process of relationships, with all the complex, messy and unsettling processes involved', they are addressing accurately this multi-piece jigsaw of human existence but this is not necessarily the best way forward for professionals delivering treatment. Writers, not health workers, are actually the best at informing us of these 'messy and unsettling processes' and George Eliot (or should we now say Mary Ann Evans) and Leo Tolstoy describe these far better that any number of professors of psychology or psychiatry.

What these new approaches with 'socially focused agendas' must do is to ally themselves with others who are expanding the scope of treatment in a more formalised way. These include those who are beginning to show that shorter treatments are likely to be at least as effective as longer ones (Laporte et al., 2018; Huxley et al., 2019; Crawford et al., 2020) and could be incorporated into a staged programme of treatment, so widening the options for treatment greatly (Paris, 2020).

It is a mistake for other practitioners of lesser status, however angry, disillusioned or despairing of their efforts, to abandon the normal rules of investigating the essential elements of new therapeutic approaches. There are indeed many models of mental disorder but it is perfectly possible to absorb these into an integrated one that accepts those that are important and discards the others that may not fit (Tyrer, 2013).

10.7 Provide Better Care for People with Personality Disorders Who Are Not Seeking Treatment

Those that do not complain do not get heard. This is true of the 90% of people who do not seek help for their personality disorders, who attend doctors much more often than others but never ask for help with their personality problems. But if doctors, and all other health professionals, ignore the presence of these problems, they will provide less good care. This has been made abundantly clear in Chapter 9, and we believe that the greater awareness that is needed will be assisted by the ICD-11 classification. The present position is that only the more severe personality disorders are being recognised in clinical practice and most of these are in people who are seeking treatment. But those with less severe disorders are having inappropriate investigations and consultations, receiving more unnecessary drug treatment, getting re-referred to many different specialists on a useless merry-go-round and provoking dissatisfaction all round by not responding as expected according to the textbooks.

One of the assets of disclosing information about personality early to patients is that at least some of these problems can be anticipated and prevented. Even if it is felt too sensitive to mention any deficiencies in personality function at a first interview, one can at least flag up possible pointers that affect treatment. One way of deflecting criticism is to ask a patient to complete a short questionnaire such as the SAPAS, SAS-PD or PASQ-11 to the patient before interview. Any of the high scoring items can then be pointed out as barriers to one type of treatment and influence the choice of an alternative.

By showing a score on a questionnaire completed at the beginning of an interview, there is no way of labelling this as a prejudiced opinion held by the practitioner. By bringing the personality status of the patient into the open, a useful dialogue is set up. So in the case of someone who is highly anxious and is determined to receive a prescription of a benzodiazepine or similar tranquilliser, the dependence risk (if present) can be pointed out from a questionnaire and the risks discussed before any decision is made.

This discussion can even be extended to people who are felt to have personality difficulty rather than disorder. So, to take another example, paroxysmal atrial fibrillation can be controlled by regular medication, but if it only occurs very occasionally and is detected immediately, medication may only be needed occasionally as required. For someone with a degree of anankastia who is very diligent at following advice, this approach may be the best one to choose.

10.8 Carry Out a Public Relations Exercise to Make Personality Disorder a Destigmatised Condition

It is very difficult to remove stigma from any condition once it has become established. So it is likely to be a long journey for the absorption of personality disorder to be placed back into the mainstream of psychiatry. The late Robert Kendell, always incisive and never dull, argued that the status and acceptability of the term 'personality disorder' would depend on whether effective treatment was available:

> If, therefore, the psychiatrists and politicians who maintain that 'antisocial personality disorder' has as good a claim to being accepted as a mental disorder as schizophrenia can demonstrate that it responds to some form of treatment that is not simply a disciplined

environment, it is likely that the opposition will melt away, and the same will be true for other types of personality disorder.

(Kendell, 2002, p. 115)

There is no doubt that successful treatments help, but despite the growth of these since Kendell's article was published the stigma of personality disorder has increased, partly because, as we have noticed earlier, of the unsatisfactory interpretations given to borderline personality disorder.

As a start, it is important for practitioners to be open about using the diagnosis, both in written reports and verbal communications. Our view is that practitioners have avoided using the label of personality disorder for three possible reasons: it is unreliable, it implies the patient is unlikable and it is deemed to be too political. All three of these are illustrated in a little snippet from John Gunn, the most prominent forensic psychiatrist of his generation. In an interview he described a meeting with a patient shortly after the UK government in 1999 had introduced the concept of dangerous and severe personality disorder:

A patient came to me and said 'I've got to stop coming to see you'. So I said 'Why?' He said, 'Well, you would have to lock me up'. I said 'What do you mean?' He said, 'I'm a personality disorder aren't I?' I said, 'I never use the term, I don't use that term in my clinic, it's not something I ever say to any patient'.

(Grounds and Gordon, 2007, p. 28)

So here we have an international expert, who sees people with personality disorder every day of his working life, saying he never uses the term, together with a patient who is so upset by the government using the term that he will stop coming to the clinic (according to Gunn, he never came again). Under these circumstances, the careful psychiatrist need not even consider stigma as, if these statements were universally true, there would be no value in ever using the diagnosis.

Many others share this concern. Freeman, although he altered his views later, in 1988 wrote that the diagnosis of personality disorder: 'tells you nothing about the patient, communicates nothing of certainty to a colleague, and predicts little about the past, present or future of the individuals' (Freeman, 1988), and Aquilina (1994, p. 306) adds 'I would suggest that the term is at best unhelpful and at worst a medicalised term of abuse.'

But we would like to think that now there are the beginnings of a shift in use and understanding. Linda Gask, a professor of psychiatry with a wide perspective, has written a very illuminating autobiography about her persistent depression and its emotional turmoil over the years (Gask, 2015). In a subsequent blog she writes:

A recent reviewer of my memoir about depression and psychiatry has noted that in describing the emotional mess of my early adult years and on-going struggles with low mood, I courageously come close to defining traits of borderline personality disorder.

I really don't mind her saying that – indeed part of me is actually surprised that she is the first person to do so. I purposefully included a description of my difficulty in relationships, mood swings and problems in trusting others alongside a description of similar problems in one of my own patients. I wanted to show not only the variety of ways that people can experience what we commonly call 'depression', but also how my own problems mirrored those of my patients, such that there was very little distance between us.

I'm well aware that there are features of my personality and behaviour that could well be called 'borderline traits' and it's interesting that no one else has mentioned this. Is it because I am a Professor of Psychiatry? Is this the kind of thing one shouldn't say to me? Most people have been incredibly supportive about my honesty, but others – including one or two mental health professional colleagues, have seemed a little embarrassed by my openness. Some will have been on the receiving end of some of my irritability and anger in the past – which is always much worse when my mood is going down. If so, I can only offer my apologies, but might add that in my experience some mental health services can be less than sufficiently understanding of the emotional problems of those whom they employ.

(Gask, 2016)

Here we see the stigma exposed. Linda is honest enough to admit that her symptoms at times were probably borderline ones but others are very reluctant to be open about this; to say this to a professor of psychiatry is close to sacrilege. What Linda is describing here are times when her personality functions were those of disorder, and her excoriating honesty about her other moods and behaviour extends to the personality spectrum also.

If there was a medical disorder that affected one in ten of the population, no matter how unpleasant, it would have to be acknowledged and be part of public discourse. The nearest equivalent to personality disorder is leprosy, not a particularly contagious disease but attracting extra prejudice because of its visual impact. It is mentioned over 50 times in the Bible and was often felt to be a curse from God, but it was never eliminated from conversation or whispered about behind cupped hands.

When public figures speak out and say that they have any disorder subject to stigma, it helps public perception and acceptance enormously. This has happened in recent years with MPs talking about their periods of depression and struggles with obsessive compulsive disorder. So we can only hope that at some point in the future, when an MP has offended another in a maladroit interchange, he might apologise by saying, 'I'm sorry for my last remark; it was just my personality difficulty getting the better of me.' Why not? It is easy to say and would bring credit on the speaker, as well as almost certainly being true.

10.9 Celebrate Personality Spectra Day on 25th May

The ICD-11 Revision Group has agreed that 25th May every year should be celebrated as International Personality Spectra Day and this is supported by many others. On this day we hope we will have events across the world that will celebrate the diversity of personality on its many spectra, one of which is the official ICD-11 classification, including all levels of severity of personality disorder. Many professional organisations in psychiatry, including the Royal College of Psychiatrists and the American Psychiatric Association, support the principles behind greater awareness of personality disorder but do not always put it directly into words. So when the American Psychiatric Association asks all psychiatrists to increase diversity by 'serving the needs of evolving, diverse, under-represented and under-served patient populations; and working to end disparities in mental health care', personality spectra should be high on their agenda.

Until then the personality disorder volcano will remain in Lisbon, welcome or unwelcome, and in all other places on the map of the world, but when everything is right, they will no longer be volcanos, just contained eruptions.

Appendices

The short scales that can be used to screen for personality disorder are listed here. Like all screening instruments, they have high sensitivity but low specificity, which means they are very good at picking up those who may have personality disorder but tend to over-identify and classify some wrongly. The list also includes one that is not listed formally – it includes a shortened version of a self-rated questionnaire for social functioning. The questionnaire has eight items, but it has been found that five of them are highly correlated with personality disorder (Moran et al., 2003).

1) Standardised Assessment of Personality – Abbreviated Scale (SAPAS)

Standardised Assessment of Personality – Abbreviated Scale (Moran et al)
Please ask your patients the following questions. Only tick a response if the patient thinks that the description applies *most of the time* and *in most situations*.
1. In general, do you have difficulty making and keeping friends? ☐**Yes** ☐No

2. Would you normally describe yourself as a loner? ☐ **Yes** ☐No
3. In general, do you trust other people? ☐Yes ☐**No** ☐
4. Do you normally lose your temper easily? **Yes** ☐No ☐
5. Are you normally an impulsive sort of person? **Yes** ☐No ☐
6. Are you normally a worrier? **Yes** ☐No
7. In general, do you depend on others a lot? ☐**Yes** ☐No
8. In general, are you a perfectionist? ☐**Yes** ☐No

Reproduced with the permission of Paul Moran.

2) Standardised Assessment of Severity of Personality Disorder (SASPD)

This questionnaire contains a series of items related to nine aspects of a person's life. For each area please could you indicate which of the four statements best describes how things are for you **in general**. We are keen to find out how things generally are for you, rather than how things might have been over recent days or weeks.

For each aspect of yourself or your life, please tick **ONE** box that best describes how you generally are.

1. Being with others
- ☐ I enjoy being with other people
- ☐ I sometimes find it difficult to be with other people
- ☐ In general, I do not like being with others
- ☐ I do not like being with other people at all and do everything to avoid them

2. Trusting other people
- ☐ I have no difficulty trusting others
- ☐ At times I find it difficult to trust others
- ☐ There are very few people I can trust
- ☐ I trust no one and this stops me from doing things I need to do

3. Friendships
- ☐ I have no difficulty making and keeping friends
- ☐ I find it difficult to make and keep friends
- ☐ I have very few friends
- ☐ I have no friends

4. Temper
- ☐ I do not lose my temper easily
- ☐ I lose my temper more easily than others
- ☐ I lose my temper easily and this gets me into difficult situations
- ☐ I lose my temper easily and this has led me to harm myself or other people

5. Acting on impulse
- ☐ I never or rarely act on impulse
- ☐ I sometimes act on impulse
- ☐ Acting on impulse gets me into trouble with others
- ☐ Acting on impulse has led me to harm myself or other people

6. Worrying

☐ In general, I am not a worrier

☐ I sometimes get worried about things that others don't

☐ I am generally a worrier

☐ Constant worrying stops me from doing things I need to do

7. Being organised

☐ It's fine with me if things are not well organised

☐ I dislike it when things are not well organised

☐ Trying to make things organised interferes with most things I need to do

☐ Trying to make things organised stops me doing everything

8. Caring about other people

☐ I care about how other people feel

☐ I don't pay much attention to whether what I do affects other people

☐ I don't care whether what I do hurts other people's feelings

☐ People say that I am 'cold blooded' or callous

9. Self-reliance

☐ I generally complete the things I need to do on my own

☐ When tackling things, I like to get help from other people

☐ When tackling things, I generally need help from other people

☐ I can't do anything by myself

Each item is scored 0 = absent, 1 = mild, 2 = moderate and 3 = severe and total score therefore ranges from 0 to 27.

The cut-off point for mild personality disorder is 8 and that for moderate personality disorder is 10. Data are not yet sufficient to indicate the cut-off point for severe personality disorder.

(From Olajide et al., 2018. Reproduced with the permission of the authors and Guilford Press, New York)

3) Personality Assessment Questionnaire for ICD-11 personality trait domains (PSQ-11) (Kim et al., 2021)

Please read the following statements and for each one, circle a number from 0 to 4 to indicate *how much this has been true for you normally*. Please circle one and only one number for every statement.

Borderline personality disorder correlates with all the above to varying degrees, so a total score of 30 or more is in the clinical range

	Statements	Never	Rarely	Some-times	Often	Always
1	How well in general do you get on with other people? (Det)	0	1	2	3	4
2	Do you normally trust them? (Det)	0	1	2	3	4
3	Do you expect the worst to happen in life? (NA)	4	3	2	1	0
4	Are you a person with high standards? (An)	0	1	2	3	4
5	Have you ever done things on impulse and regretted them afterward? (Dis)	0	1	2	3	4
6	Do you plan everything in detail in life? (An)	0	1	2	3	4
7	Do people ever say you are too fussy or conscientious, or even a perfectionist? (An)	0	1	2	3	4
8	Do you have any really close relationships? (Det)	4	3	2	1	0
9	Do you care about other people? (Dis)	4	3	2	1	0
10	Do you feel gloomier about the future than most other people? (NA)	0	1	2	3	4

	Statements	Never	Rarely	Some-times	Often	Always
11	Do you ever do things on the spur of the moment without caring about the consequences? (Dis)	0	1	2	3	4
12	Do you lack self-confidence? (NA)	0	1	2	3	4
13	Do you tend to manipulate others to get what you want in life? (Dissoc)	0	1	2	3	4
14	Are you normally a fussy person? (An)	0	1	2	3	4
15	Do you ever worry about things that most people would not be concerned about? (NA)	0	1	2	3	4
16	Are you more nervous than most other people? (NA)	0	1	2	3	4
17	Are you a person who likes to stay apart from other people? (Det)	0	1	2	3	4

Key: An = Anankastia, Det = Detachment, Dis = Disinhibition, Dissoc = Dissocial, NA = Negative affectivity
The threshold for each of these domains has yet to be determined, but the following total scores suggest the domain requirements have been met:
Anankastia: 9
Detachment: 7
Disinhibition: 4
Dissociality: 4
Negative affectivity: 10

4) Short Social Functioning Questionnaire (SSFQ) (Tyrer et al., 2021)

Please look at the statements below and tick the reply that comes closest to how you have been generally.

A score of 7 or more is suggestive of personality difficulty or disorder.

I complete my tasks at work and home satisfactorily.	Most of the time	☐	0
	Quite often	☐	1
	Sometimes	☐	2
	Not at all	☐	3
I find my tasks at work and at home very stressful.	Most of the time	☐	3
	Quite often	☐	2
	Sometimes	☐	1
	Not at all	☐	0
I have difficulties in getting and keeping close relationships.	Severe difficulties	☐	3
	Some problems	☐	2
	Occasional problems	☐	1
	No problems at all	☐	0
I have problems in my sex life.	Severe problems	☐	3
	Moderate problems	☐	2
	Occasional problems	☐	1
	No problems at all	☐	0

(cont.)

I feel lonely and isolated from other people.	Almost all the time	☐	3
	Much of the time		
	Not usually	☐	2
	Not at all		
		☐	1
		☐	0

I enjoy my spare time.	Very much	☐	0
	Sometimes		
	Not often	☐	1
	Not at all		
		☐	2
		☐	3

References

A-Tjak, J. G. L., Davis, M. L., Morina, N., Powers, M. B., Smits, J. A. J. & Emmelkamp, P. M. G. (2015). A meta-analysis of the efficacy of Acceptance and Commitment Therapy for clinically relevant mental and physical health problems. *Psychotherapy and Psychosomatics*, 84(1),30–6. doi:10.1159/000365764

Abraham, P. F. & Calabrese, J. R. (2008). Evidenced-based pharmacologic treatment of borderline personality disorder: A shift from SSRIs to anticonvulsants and atypical antipsychotics? *Journal of Affective Disorders*, 111(1),21–30. doi:10.1016/j.jad.2008.01.024

Adams, H. E., Feuerstein, M. & Fowler, J. L. (1980). Migraine headache: Review of parameters, etiology, and intervention. *Psychological Bulletin*, 87(2),217–37. doi:10.1037/0033-2909.87.2.217

Akiskal, H. S., Hirschfeld, R. M. A. & Yerevanian, B. I. (1983). The relationship of personality to affective disorders: A critical review. *Archives of General Psychiatry*, 40 (7),801–10. doi:10.1001/archpsyc.1983.01790060099013

Akiskal, H. S. & Mckinney, W. T., Jr (1973). Depressive disorders: Toward a unified hypothesis. *Science*, 182(4107),20–9. doi:10.1126/science.182.4107.20

Alden, L. E. & Capreol, M. J. (1993). Avoidant personality disorder: Interpersonal problems as predictors of treatment response. *Behavior Therapy*, 24(3),357–76. doi:10.1016/S0005-7894(05)80211-4

Aldington, R. (ed.) (1924). *A Book of 'Characters' from Theophrastus: Joseph Hall, Sir Thomas Overbury, Nicolas Breton, John Earle, Thomas Fuller, and Other English Authors; Jean De La Bruyere, Vauvenargues, and Other French Authors*, London, Routledge.

Allport, G. W. (1927). Concepts of trait and personality. *Psychological Bulletin*, 24 (5),284–93. doi:10.1037/h0073629

Allport, F. H. & Allport, G. W. (1921). Personality traits: Their classification and measurement. *The Journal of Abnormal Psychology and Social Psychology*, 16(1),6–40. doi:10.1037/h0069790

American Psychiatric Association (1980). *Diagnostic and Statistical Manual of Mental Disorders DSM-III* (3rd ed.), Washington, DC, American Psychiatric Association.

American Psychiatric Association Practice Guidelines (2001). Practice guideline for the treatment of patients with borderline personality disorder. American Psychiatric Association. *American Journal of Psychiatry*, 158(10 Suppl),1–52.

Andrews, G. (1996). Comorbidity and the general neurotic syndrome. *British Journal of Psychiatry*, 168 (Supplement 30),76–84.

Andrews, G., Stewart, G., Morris-Yates, A., Holt, P. & Henderson, S. (1990). Evidence for a general neurotic syndrome. *British Journal of Psychiatry*, 157, 6–12.

Aquilina, C. (1994). Label of personality disorder [Correspondence]. *Psychiatric Bulletin*, 18(5),305–6.

Aviram, R. B., Brodsky, B. S. & Stanley, B. (2006). Borderline personality disorder, stigma, and treatment implications. *Harvard Review of Psychiatry*, 14(5),249–56. doi:10.1080/10673220600975121

Bach, B. & Bernstein, D. P. (2019). Schema therapy conceptualization of personality functioning and traits in ICD-11 and DSM-5. *Current Opinion in Psychiatry*, 32(1),38–49. doi:10.1097/YCO.0000000000000464

Bach, B., Christensen, S., Kongerslev, M. T., Sellbom, M. & Simonsen, E. (2020a). Structure of clinician-reported ICD-11 personality disorder trait qualifiers. *Psychological Assessment*, 32(1),50–9. doi:10.1037/pas0000747

Bach, B. & First, M. B. (2018). Application of the ICD-11 classification of personality disorders. *BMC Psychiatry*, 18(1),351. doi:10.1186/s12888-018-1908-3

Bach, B., Kerber, A., Aluja, A., Bastiaens, T., Keeley, J. W., Claes, L., et al. (2020b). International assessment of DSM-5 and ICD-11 personality disorder traits: Toward a common nosology in DSM-5.1. *Psychopathology*, 53(3–4),179–88. doi:10.1159/000507589

Bach, B. & Presnall-Shvorin, J. (2020). Using DSM-5 and ICD-11 personality traits in clinical treatment. In Lejuez, C. & Gratz, K. (eds.) *The Cambridge Handbook of Personality Disorders*, Cambridge, Cambridge University Press.

Bach, B., Sellbom, M., Kongerslev, M., Simonsen, E., Krueger, R. F. & Mulder, R. T. (2017). Deriving ICD-11 personality disorder domains from DSM-5 traits: Initial attempt to harmonize two diagnostic systems. *Acta Psychiatrica Scandinavica*, 136(1),108–17. doi:10.1111/acps.12748

Bach, B., Sellbom, M., Skjernov, M. & Simonsen, E. (2018). ICD-11 and DSM-5 personality trait domains capture categorical personality disorders: Finding a common ground. *Australian and New Zealand Journal of Psychiatry*, 52(5),425–34. doi:10.1177/0004867417727867

Bach, B. & Simonsen, S. (2021). How does level of personality functioning inform clinical management and treatment? Implications for ICD-11 classification of personality disorder severity. *Current Opinion in Psychiatry*, 34(1),54–63. doi:10.1097/YCO.0000000000000658

Bagby, R. M., Gralnick, T. M., Al-Dajani, N. & Uliaszek, A. A. (2016). The role of the five-factor model in personality assessment and treatment planning. *Clinical Psychology: Science and Practice*, 23(4),365–81. doi:10.1111/cpsp.12175

Baleydier, B., Damsa, C., Schutzbach, C., Stauffer, O. & Glauser, D. (2003). Étude comparative des caractéristiques sociodémographiques et des facteurs prédictifs de soins de patients Suisses et étrangers consultant un service d'urgences psychiatriques [Comparison between Swiss and foreign patients characteristics at the psychiatric emergencies department and the

predictive factors of their management strategies]. *Encephale*, 29(3 Pt 1),205–12. doi: ENC-6-2003-29-3-0013-7006-101019-ART2

Bangash, A. (2020). Personality disorders in later life: Epidemiology, presentation and management. *BJPsych Advances*, 26(4),208–18. doi:10.1192/bja.2020.16

Barlow, D. H., Farchione, T. J., Fairholme, C. P., et al. (2011). *Unified Protocol for Transdiagnostic Treatment of Emotional Disorders: Therapist Guide*, New York, Oxford University Press.

Barnicot, K. & Crawford, M. (2019). Dialectical behaviour therapy v. mentalisation-based therapy for borderline personality disorder. *Psychological Medicine*, 49(12),2060–8. doi:10.1017/S0033291718002878

Barnicot, K., Gonzalez, R., McCabe, R. & Priebe, S. (2016). Skills use and common treatment processes in dialectical behaviour therapy for borderline personality disorder. *Journal of Behavior Therapy and Experimental Psychiatry*, 52, 147–56. doi:10.1016/j.jbtep.2016.04.006

Barrash, J., Kroll, J., Carey, K. & Sines, L. (1983). Discriminating borderline disorder from other personality disorders: Cluster analysis of the diagnostic interview for borderlines. *Archives of General Psychiatry*, 40(12),1297–302. doi:10.1001/archpsyc.1983.01790110039008

Barry, D. T., Cutter, C. J., Beitel, M., Kerns, R. D., Liong, C. & Schottenfeld, R. S. (2016). Psychiatric disorders among patients seeking treatment for co-occurring chronic pain and opioid use disorder. *Journal of Clinical Psychiatry*, 77(10),1413–19. doi:10.4088/JCP.15m09963

Bateman, A. W. (2011). Throwing the baby out with the bathwater? [Commentary]. *Personality and Mental Health*, 5(4),274–80. doi:10.1002/pmh.184

Bateman, A. & Fonagy, P. (1999a). Effectiveness of partial hospitalization in the treatment of borderline personality disorder: A randomized controlled trial. *American Journal of Psychiatry* 156(10),1563–9. doi:10.1176/ajp.156.10.1563

Bateman, A. W. & Fonagy, P. (1999b). Psychotherapy for severe personality disorder: Article did not do justice to available research data [Letter to the Editor]. *BMJ*, 319 (7211),709–10;author reply 710–1. doi:10.1136/bmj.319.7211.709a

Bateman, A. & Fonagy, P. (2009). Randomized controlled trial of outpatient mentalization-based treatment versus structured clinical management for borderline personality disorder. *American Journal of Psychiatry*, 166(12),1355–64. doi:10.1176/appi.ajp.2009.09040539

Bateman, A. & Fonagy, P. (2013). Impact of clinical severity on outcomes of mentalisation-based treatment for borderline personality disorder. *British Journal of Psychiatry*, 203(3),221–7. doi:10.1192/bjp. bp.112.121129

Bateman, A. & Fonagy, P. (2016). *Mentalization-Based Treatment for Personality Disorders: A Practical Guide*, New York, Oxford University Press.

Bateman, A. W. & Krawitz, R. (2013). *Borderline Personality Disorder: An Evidence-Based Guide for Generalist Mental Health Professionals*, Oxford, Oxford University Press.

Beck, A. T., Davis, D. D. & Freeman, A. (2015). *Cognitive Therapy of Personality Disorders* (3rd ed.), New York, Guilford Press.

Beck, A. T., Freeman, A. & Associates. (1990). *Cognitive Therapy of Personality Disorders*, New York, Guilford Press.

Behary, W. T. & Dieckman, E. (2012). Schema therapy for narcissism: The art of empathic confrontation, limit-setting, and leverage. In Campbell, W. K. & Miller, J. D. (eds.) *The Handbook of Narcissism and Narcissistic Personality Disorder: Theoretical Approaches, Empirical Findings, and Treatments.* New York, John Wiley & Sons.

Bender, D. S., Morey, L. C. & Skodol, A. E. (2011). Toward a model for assessing level of personality functioning in DSM-5, Part I: A review of theory and methods. *Journal of Personality Assessment*, 93(4),332–46. doi:10.1080/00223891.2011.583808

Benefield, N. & Haigh, R. (2020). Personality disorder: Breakdown in the relational field. In Ramsden, J., Prince, S. & Blazdell, J. (eds.) *Working Effectively with 'Personality Disorder': Contemporary and Critical Approaches to Clinical and Organizational Practice*. London, Luminate (Pavilion Publishing and Media Ltd).

Benefield, N., Turner, K., Bolger, L. & Bainbridge, C. (2017). Psychologically informed planned environments: A new optimism for criminal justice provision? In Akerman, G., Needs, A. & Bainbridge, C. (eds.) *Transforming Environments and Rehabilitation: A Guide for Practitioners in Forensic Settings and Criminal Justice.* 1st ed. London, Routledge.

Bernstein, D. P., Arntz, A. & De Vos, M. (2007a). Schema focused therapy in forensic settings: Theoretical model and recommendations for best clinical practice. *International Journal of Forensic Mental Health*, 6(2),169–83. doi:10.1080/14999013.2007.10471261

Bernstein, D. P., Iscan, C., Maser, J., Board of Directors of the Association for Research in Personality Disorders & Board of Directors of the International Society for the Study of Personality Disorders (2007b). Opinions of personality disorder experts regarding the DSM-IV personality disorders classification system. *Journal of Personality Disorders*, 21 (5),536–51. doi:10.1521/pedi.2007.21.5.536

Bickerdike, L., Booth, A., Wilson, P. M., Farley, K. & Wright, K. (2017). Social prescribing: less rhetoric and more reality. A systematic review of the evidence. *BMJ Open*, 7(4), e013384. doi:10.1136/bmjopen-2016-013384

Bion, W. R. & Rickman, J. (1943). Intra-group tensions in therapy: Their study as the task of the group. *Lancet*, 242(6274),678–82. doi:10.1016/S0140-6736(00)88231-8

Black, D. W. (2013). *Bad Boys, Bad Men: Confronting Antisocial Personality Disorder (Sociopathy)* (2nd ed.), Oxford, Oxford University Press.

Black, D. W., Baumgard, C. H. & Bell, S. E. (1995). A 16- to 45-year follow-up of 71 men with antisocial personality disorder. *Comprehensive Psychiatry*, 36(2),130–40. doi:10.1016/s0010-440x(95)90108-6

Bleidorn, W. & Ködding, C. (2013). The divided self and psychological (mal) adjustment – A meta-analytic review. *Journal of Research in*

Personality, 47(5),547–52. doi:10.1016/j.jrp.2013.04.009

Blum, N., St John, D., Pfohl, B., et al. (2008). Systems Training for Emotional Predictability and Problem Solving (STEPPS) for outpatients with borderline personality disorder: A randomized controlled trial and 1-year follow-up. *American Journal of Psychiatry*, 165(4),468–78. doi:10.1176/appi.ajp.2007.07071079

Bogdanowicz, K. M., Stewart, R., Broadbent, M., et al. (2015). Double trouble: Psychiatric comorbidity and opioid addiction – all-cause and cause-specific mortality. *Drug Alcohol Depend*, 148, 85–92. doi:10.1016/j.drugalcdep.2014.12.025

Bowen, M. L. (2016). Stigma: Content analysis of the representation of people with personality disorder in the UK popular press, 2001–2012. *International Journal of Mental Health Nursing*, 25(6),598–605. doi:10.1111/inm.12213

Braden, J. B. & Sullivan, M. D. (2008). Suicidal thoughts and behavior among adults with self-reported pain conditions in the national comorbidity survey replication. *The Journal of Pain*, 9(12),1106–15. doi:10.1016/j.jpain.2008.06.004

Brazão, N., Rijo, D., Salvador, M. D. C. & Pinto-Gouveia, J. (2018). The efficacy of the growing pro-social program in reducing anger, shame, and paranoia over time in male prison inmates: A randomized controlled trial. *Journal of Research in Crime and Delinquency*, 55(5),649–86. doi:10.1177/0022427818782733

British Medical Association & Royal Pharmaceutical Society of Great Britain (2010). *British National Formulary (BNF) 59* (59th ed.), London, Pharmaceutical Press.

British Psychological Society. (n.d.). *Introduction to the PTMF* [Online]. Available: https://www.bps.org.uk/power-threat-meaning-framework/introduction-ptmf [Accessed 25 February 2021].

Buer Christensen, T., Eikenaes, I., Hummelen, B., et al. (2020). Level of personality functioning as a predictor of psychosocial functioning – Concurrent validity of criterion A. *Personality Disorders:*

Theory, Research, and Treatment, 11 (2),79–90. doi:10.1037/per0000352

Burton, R. (1621; republished 1927). *The Anatomy of Melancholy*, New York, George H. Doran Company.

Buss, D. M. & Penke, L. (2015). Evolutionary personality psychology. In Mikulincer, M., Shaver, P. R., Cooper, M. L. & Larsen, R. J. (eds.) *APA Handbook of Personality and Social Psychology: Personality Processes and Individual Differences*. Washington, DC, American Psychological Association.

Caldwell-Harris, C. L. & Ayçiçegi, A. (2006). When personality and culture clash: The psychological distress of allocentrics in an individualist culture and idiocentrics in a collectivist culture. *Transcultural Psychiatry*, 43(3),331–61. doi:10.1177/1363461506066982

Calliess, I. T., Sieberer, M., Machleidt, W. & Ziegenbein, M. (2008). Personality disorders in a cross-cultural perspective: Impact of culture and migration on diagnosis and etiological aspects. *Current Psychiatry Reviews*, 4(1),39–41. doi:10.2174/157340008783743776

Campbell, G., Bruno, R., Darke, S. & Degenhardt, L. (2015). Associations of borderline personality with pain, problems with medications and suicidality in a community sample of chronic non-cancer pain patients prescribed opioids for pain. *General Hospital Psychiatry*, 37(5),434–40. doi:10.1016/j.genhosppsych.2015.05.004

Cantor-Graae, E. & Selten, J. P. (2005). Schizophrenia and migration: A meta-analysis and review. *American Journal of Psychiatry*, 162(1),12–24. doi:10.1176/appi.ajp.162.1.12

Carnovale, M., Carlson, E. N., Quilty, L. C. & Bagby, R. M. (2019). Discrepancies in self- and informant-reports of personality pathology: Examining the DSM–5 Section III trait model. *Personality Disorders: Theory, Research, and Treatment*, 10(5),456–67. doi:10.1037/per0000342

Caspi, A., Roberts, B. W. & Shiner, R. L. (2005). Personality development: Stability and change. *Annual Review of Psychology*, 56,

453–84. doi:10.1146/annurev. psych.55.090902.141913

Chamberlain, S. R., Stochl, J., Redden, S. A. & Grant, J. E. (2018). Latent traits of impulsivity and compulsivity: Toward dimensional psychiatry. *Psychological Medicine*, 48 (5),810–21. doi:10.1017/S0033291717002185

Chanen, A. M., Jackson, H. J., McCutcheon, L. K., et al. (2008). Early intervention for adolescents with borderline personality disorder using cognitive analytic therapy: Randomised controlled trial. *British Journal of Psychiatry* 193(6),477–84. doi:10.1192/bjp.bp.107.048934

Chanen, A. M. & McCutcheon, L. (2013). Prevention and early intervention for borderline personality disorder: Current status and recent evidence. *British Journal of Psychiatry*, 202(S54),S24–9. doi:10.1192/bjp. bp.112.119180

Chaplin, S. (2018). Consensus statement calls for better treatment for personality disorder. *Progress in Neurology and Psychiatry* (Wiley). Available: https://www.progressnp.com/new s/consensus-statement-calls-better-treatment-personality-disorder/ [Last accessed 11 February 2021].

Chartonas, D., Kyratsous, M., Dracass, S., Lee, T. & Bhui, K. (2017). Personality disorder: Still the patients psychiatrists dislike? *BJPsych Bulletin*, 41(1),12–17. doi:10.1192/pb. bp.115.052456

Chen, C. & Stevenson, H. W. (1995). Motivation and mathematics achievement: A comparative study of Asian-American, Caucasian-American, and East Asian high school students. *Child Development*, 66 (4),1214–34. doi:10.2307/1131808

Cheung, F. M., Cheung, S. F., Leung, K., Ward, C. & Leong, F. (2003). The English Version of the Chinese Personality Assessment Inventory. *Journal of Cross-Cultural Psychology*, 34(4),433–52. doi:10.1177/0022022103034004004

Church, A. T. (2016). Personality traits across cultures. *Current Opinion in Psychology*, 8, 22–30. doi:10.1016/j.copsyc.2015.09.014

Church, A. T. (2020). Culture and personality: Toward an integrated cultural trait

psychology. *Journal of Personality*, 68 (4),651–703. doi:10.1111/1467-6494.00112

Clark, L. A., Livesley, W. J. & Morey, L. (1997). Special feature: Personality disorder assessment: The challenge of construct validity. *Journal of Personality Disorders*, 11 (3),205–31. doi:10.1521/pedi.1997.11.3.205

Clark, L. A., Nuzum, H. & Ro, E. (2018). Manifestations of personality impairment severity: Comorbidity, course/prognosis, psychosocial dysfunction, and 'borderline' personality features. *Current Opinion in Psychology*, 21, 117–21. doi:10.1016/j. copsyc.2017.12.004

Clarkin, J. F., Levy, K. N., Lenzenweger, M. F. & Kernberg, O. F. (2007). Evaluating three treatments for borderline personality disorder: A multiwave study. *American Journal of Psychiatry*, 164(6),922–8. doi:10.1176/appi.ajp.164.6.922

Clarkin, J. F., Yeomans, F. E. & Kernberg, O. E. (1999). *Psychotherapy for Borderline Personality*, New York, John Wiley & Sons.

Cleckley, H. M. (1941). *The Mask of Sanity: An Attempt to Reinterpret the So-Called Psychopathic Personality* (1st ed.), St Louis, MO, Mosby.

Cleckley, H. M. (1988). *The Mask of Sanity: An Attempt to Clarify Some Issues around the So-Called Psychopathic Personality* (5th ed.), Augusta, Emily S. Cleckley.

Cohen, B. J., Nestadt, G., Samuels, J. F., Romanoski, A. J., Mchugh, P. R. & Rabins, P. V. (1994). Personality disorder in later life: A community study. *British Journal of Psychiatry*, 165(4),493–9. doi:10.1192/ bjp.165.4.493

Coid, J., Yang, M., Tyrer, P., Roberts, A. & Ullrich, S. (2006). Prevalence and correlates of personality disorder in Great Britain. *British Journal of Psychiatry*, 188(5),423–31. doi:10.1192/bjp.188.5.423

Compton, W. M., 3rd., Helzer, J. E., Hwu, H. G., et al. (1991). New methods in cross-cultural psychiatry: Psychiatric illness in Taiwan and the United States. *American Journal of Psychiatry*, 148(12),1697–704. doi:10.1176/ ajp.148.12.1697

Conway, C. C., Hammen, C. & Brennan, P. A. (2016). Optimizing prediction of psychosocial and clinical outcomes with a transdiagnostic model of personality disorder. *Journal of Personality Disorders*, 30 (4),545–66. doi:10.1521/pedi_2015_29_218

Cooke, D. J. (1996). Psychopathic personality in different cultures: What do we know? What do we need to find out? *Journal of Personality Disorders*, 10(1),23–40. doi:10.1521/pedi.1996.10.1.23

Crawford, M. J., Koldobsky, N., Mulder, R. T. & Tyrer, P. (2011). Classifying personality disorder according to severity. *Journal of Personality Disorders*, 25(3),321–30. doi:10.1521/pedi.2011.25.3.321

Crawford, M. J., Sanatinia, R., Barrett, B., et al. (2018). The clinical effectiveness and cost-effectiveness of lamotrigine in borderline personality disorder: A randomized placebo-controlled trial. *American Journal of Psychiatry*, 175(8),756–64. doi:10.1176/appi.ajp.2018.17091006

Crawford, M. J., Thana, L., Parker, J., et al. (2020). Structured Psychological Support for people with personality disorder: Feasibility randomised controlled trial of a low-intensity intervention. *BJPsych Open*, 6(2), e25. doi:10.1192/bjo.2020.7

Cristea, I. A., Gentili, C., Cotet, C. D., Palomba, D., Barbui, C. & Cuijpers, P. (2017). Efficacy of psychotherapies for borderline personality disorder: A systematic review and meta-analysis. *JAMA Psychiatry*, 74(4),319–28. doi:10.1001/jamapsychiatry.2016.4287

Dahl, A. A. (1986). Some aspects of the DSM-III personality disorders illustrated by a consecutive sample of hospitalized patients. *Acta Psychiatrica Scandinavica*, 73, 61–7. doi:10.1111/j.1600-0447.1986.tb10526.x

Davidson, K. (2007). *Cognitive Therapy for Personality Disorders: A Guide for Clinicians*, London, Routledge.

Davidson, K., Norrie, J., Tyrer, P., et al. (2006). The effectiveness of cognitive behavior therapy for borderline personality disorder: Results from the borderline personality disorder study of cognitive therapy (BOSCOT) trial. *Journal of Personality Disorders*, 20(5),450–65. doi:10.1521/pedi.2006.20.5.450

Davidson, K. M., Tyrer, P., Norrie, J., Palmer, S. J. & Tyrer, H. (2010). Cognitive therapy v. usual treatment for borderline personality disorder: Prospective 6-year follow-up. *British Journal of Psychiatry*, 197 (6),456–62. doi:10.1192/bjp.bp.109.074286

Davidson, K. M., Tyrer, P., Tata, P., et al. (2009). Cognitive behaviour therapy for violent men with antisocial personality disorder in the community: An exploratory randomized controlled trial. *Psychological Medicine*, 39 (4),569–77. doi:10.1017/S0033291708004066

De Aquino Ferreira, L. F., Queiroz Pereira, F. H., Neri Benevides, A. & Aguiar Melo, M. C. (2018). Borderline personality disorder and sexual abuse: A systematic review. *Psychiatry Research*, 262, 70–7. doi:10.1016/j.psychres.2018.01.043

De Fruyt, F. & De Clercq, B. (2014). Antecedents of personality disorder in childhood and adolescence: Toward an integrative developmental model. *Annual Review of Clinical Psychology*, 10, 449–476. doi:10.1146/annurev-clinpsy-032813-153634

Distel, M. A., Carlier, A., Middeldorp, C. M., Derom, C. A., Lubke, G. H. & Boomsma, D. I. (2011). Borderline personality traits and adult attention-deficit hyperactivity disorder symptoms: A genetic analysis of comorbidity. *American Journal of Medical Genetics Part B*, 156(7),817–25. doi:10.1002/ajmg.b.31226

De Lacy, N. & King, B. H. (2013). Revisiting the relationship between autism and schizophrenia: Toward an integrated neurobiology. *Annual Review of Clinical Psychology*, 9, 555–587.

Doering, S., Horz, S., Rentrop, M., et al. (2010). Transference-focused psychotherapy v. treatment by community psychotherapists for borderline personality disorder: Randomised controlled trial. *British Journal of Psychiatry*, 196(5),389–95. doi:10.1192/bjp.bp.109.070177

Dowson, J. H. & Berrios, G. E. (1991). Factor structure of DSM-III-R personality disorders shown by self-report questionnaire: Implications for classifying and assessing personality disorders. *Acta Psychiatrica*

Scandinavica, 84(6),555–60. doi:10.1111/ j.1600-0447.1991.tb03194.x

Drake, M. M., Morris, M. & Davis, T. J. (2017). Neuroticism's susceptibility to distress: Moderated with mindfulness. *Personality and Individual Differences*, 106, 248–52. doi:10.1016/j.paid.2016.10.060

Duggan, C., Sham, P., Lee, A. & Minne, C. (1996). Neuroticism: A vulnerability marker for depression evidence from a family study. *Journal of Affective Disorders*, 35, 139–43.

Duggan, C., Huband, N., Smailagic, N., Ferriter, M. & Adams, C. (2008). The use of pharmacological treatments for people with personality disorder: A systematic review of randomized controlled trials. *Personality and Mental Health*, 2(3),119–70. doi:10.1002/ pmh.41

Duggan, C., Parry, G., Mcmurran, M., Davidson, K. & Dennis, J. (2014). The recording of adverse events from psychological treatments in clinical trials: Evidence from a review of NIHR-funded trials. *Trials*, 15, 335. doi:10.1186/1745-6215-15-335

Eagles, J. (2017). *Starting to Shrink*, London, Austin Macauley.

Eaton, N. R. & Greene, A. L. (2018). Personality disorders: Community prevalence and socio-demographic correlates. *Current Opinion in Psychology*, 21, 28–32. doi:10.1016/j.copsyc.2017.09.001

Ekselius, L., Lindström, E., Von Knorring, L., Bodlund, O. & Kullgren, G. (1994). SCID II interviews and the SCID Screen questionnaire as diagnostic tools for personality disorders in DSM-III-R. *Acta Psychiatrica Scandinavica*, 90(2),120–3. doi:10.1111/j.1600-0447.1994.tb01566.x

Emmelkamp, P. M. G., Benner, A., Kuipers, A., Feiertag, G. A., Koster, H. C. & Van Apeldoorn, F. J. (2006). Comparison of brief dynamic and cognitive-behavioural therapies in avoidant personality disorder. *British Journal of Psychiatry*, 189(1),60–4. doi:10.1192/bjp.bp.105.012153

Emmelkamp, P. M. G. & Meyerbröker, K. (2020). *Personality Disorders* (2nd ed.), London, Psychological Press.

Engels, G. I., Duijsens, I. J., Haringsma, R. & Van Putten, C. M. (2003). Personality disorders in the elderly compared to four younger age groups: A cross-sectional study of community residents and mental health patients. *Journal of Personality Disorders*, 17 (5),447–59. doi:10.1521/pedi.17.5.447.22971

English, T. & Chen, S. (2011). Self-concept consistency and culture: The differential impact of two forms of consistency. *Personality and Social Psychology Bulletin*, 37 (6),838–49. doi:10.1177/0146167211400621

Eurelings-Bontekoe, E. H., Van Dam, A., Luyten, P., et al. (2009). Structural personality organization as assessed with theory driven profile interpretation of the Dutch short form of the MMPI predicts dropout and treatment response in brief cognitive behavioral group therapy for axis I disorders. *Journal of Personality Assessment*, 91(5),439–452. doi:10.1080/ 00223890903087927

Eysenck, H. J. (1970). The classification of depressive illnesses. *British Journal of Psychiatry*, 117(538),241–50. doi:10.1192/ S0007125000193195

Eysenck, H. J. & Eysenck, S. B. G. (1975). *Manual of the Eysenck Personality Questionnaire*, London, Hodder & Stoughton.

Fabrega, H., Jr. (1994). Personality disorders as medical entities: A cultural interpretation. *Journal of Personality Disorders*, 8(2),149–67. doi:10.1521/pedi.1994.8.2.149

Faiad, Y., Khoury, B., Daouk, S., et al. (2018). Frequency of use of the International Classification of Diseases ICD-10 diagnostic categories for mental and behavioural disorders across world regions. *Epidemiology and Psychiatric Sciences*, 27, 568–76.

Farstad, S. M., McGeown, L. M. & Von Ranson, K. M. (2016). Eating disorders and personality, 2004–2016: A systematic review and meta-analysis. *Clinical Psychology Review*, 46, 91–105. doi:10.1016/j. cpr.2016.04.005

Fava, M., Bouffides, E., Pava, J. A., McCarthy, M. K., Steingard, R. J. & Rosenbaum, J. F. (1994). Personality disorder comorbidity with major depression and response to fluoxetine treatment. *Psychotherapy and Psychosomatics*, 62(3–4),160–7. doi:10.1159/000288918

Feinstein, A. R. (1970). The pre-therapeutic classification of co-morbidity in chronic disease. *Journal of Chronic Diseases*, 23 (7),455–68. doi:10.1016/0021-9681(70)90054-8

Ferguson, E. (2013). Personality is of central concern to understand health: Towards a theoretical model for health psychology. *Health Psychology Review*, 7(Suppl 1), S32–70. doi:10.1080/17437199.2010.547985

Fischer, C. T. & Finn, S. E. (2008). Developing the life meaning of psychological test data: Collaborative and therapeutic approaches. In Archer, R. P. & Smith, S. R. (eds.) *Personality Assessment*. New York, Routledge.

Fok, M., Hayes, R. D., Chang, C. K., Stewart, R., Callard, F. J. & Moran, P. (2012). Life expectancy at birth and all-cause mortality among people with personality disorder. *Journal of Psychosomatic Research*, 73 (2),104–7. doi:10.1016/j.jpsychores.2012.05.001

Fok, M., Hotopf, M., Stewart, R., Hatch, S., Hayes, R. & Moran, P. (2014). Personality disorder and self-rated health: A population-based cross-sectional survey. *Journal of Personality Disorders*, 28(3),319–33. doi:10.1521/pedi_2013_27_119

Foulds, J. A., Boden, J. M., Newton-Howes, G. M., Mulder, R. T. & Horwood, L. J. (2017). The role of novelty seeking as a predictor of substance use disorder outcomes in early adulthood. *Addiction*, 112 (9),1629–37. doi:10.1111/add.13838

Foulkes, S. H. (1946). Group analysis in a military neurosis centre. *Lancet*, 247 (6392),303–6.

Frances, A. (2013). *Saving Normal: An Insider's Revolt against Out-of-Control Psychiatric Diagnosis, DSM-5, Big Pharma, and the Medicalization of Ordinary Life*, New York, William Morrow.

Freeman, C. (1988). Personality disorders. In Kendell, R. E. & Zealley, A. K. (eds.) *Companion Guide to Psychiatric Studies*. 4th ed. Edinburgh, Churchill Livingstone.

Freud, S. (1916; republished 1963). Introductory Lectures on Psycho-Analysis (Parts I and II) (1915–1916). In Strachey, J., Freud, A., Strachey, A. & Tyson, A. (eds.) *The Standard Edition of the Complete Psychological Works of Sigmund Freud*. London, Hogarth Press.

Freud, S. (1925). On narcissism: An introduction (1914). In Strachey, J. (ed.) *The Standard Edition of the Complete Psychological Works of Sigmund Freud*. London, Hogarth Press.

Friborg, O., Martinsen, E. W., Martinussen, M., Kaiser, S., Øvergård, K. T. & Rosenvinge, J. H. (2014). Comorbidity of personality disorders in mood disorders: A meta-analytic review of 122 studies from 1988 to 2010. *Journal of Affective Disorders*, 152–154, 1–11. doi:10.1016/j.jad.2013.08.023

Friborg, O., Martinussen, M., Kaiser, S., Øvergård, K. T. & Rosenvinge, J. H. (2013). Comorbidity of personality disorders in anxiety disorders: A meta-analysis of 30 years of research. *Journal of Affective Disorders*, 145 (2),143–55. doi:10.1016/j.jad.2012.07.004

Friedman, H. S. & Booth-Kewley, S. (1987). The 'disease-prone personality'. A meta-analytic view of the construct. *The American Psychologist*, 42(6),539–55. doi:10.1037//0003-066x.42.6.539

Friedman, H. S. & Kern, M. L. (2014). Personality, well-being, and health. *Annual Review of Psychology*, 65(1),719–42. doi:10.1146/annurev-psych-010213-115123

Frost, R., Hyland, P., Shevlin, M. & Murphy, J. (2020). Distinguishing complex PTSD from borderline personality disorder among individuals with a history of sexual trauma: A latent class analysis. *European Journal of Trauma & Dissociation*, 4(1),100080. doi:10.1016/j.ejtd.2018.08.004

Fry, S. (2018). Foreword. In Tyrer, P. (ed.) *Taming the Beast Within: Shredding the Stereotypes of Personality Disorder*. London, Sheldon Press.

Fyer, M. R., Frances, A. J., Sullivan, T., Hurt, S. W. & Clarkin, J. (1988). Comorbidity of borderline personality disorder. *Archives of General Psychiatry*, 45(4),348–52. doi:10.1001/archpsyc.1988.01800280060008

Galen (2019). *De Temperamentis.* Edited and translated by P. N. Singer, P. J van der Eijk & P. Tassinari. Cambridge, Cambridge University Press.

Gardiner, C., Tsukagoshi, S., Nur, U. & Tyrer, P. (2010). Associations of treatment resisting (Type R) and treatment seeking (Type S) personalities in medical students. *Personality and Mental Health*, 4(2),59–63. doi:10.1002/pmh.106

Gask, L. (2015). *The Other Side of Silence: A Psychiatrist's Memoir of Depression,* Chichester, UK, Vie Books (Summersdale).

Gask, L. (4 March 2016). Borderline Traits. *Patching the Soul* [Online]. Available from: https://lindagask.com/2016/03/04/border line-traits/ [Accessed 12 February 2021].

Gaudio, S. & Dakanalis, A. (2018). Personality and eating and weight disorders: An open research challenge. *Eating and Weight Disorders*, 23(2),143–7. doi:10.1007/s40519-017-0463-0

Giesen-Bloo, J., Van Dyck, R., Spinhoven, et al. (2006). Outpatient psychotherapy for borderline personality disorder: Randomized trial of schema-focused therapy vs transference-focused psychotherapy. *Archives of General Psychiatry*, 63(6),649–58. doi:10.1001/archpsyc.63.6.649

Gilbert, P. (2014). The origins and nature of compassion focused therapy. *British Journal of Clinical Psychology*, 53(1),6–41. doi:0.1111/bjc.12043

Gilbert, P. & Procter, S. (2006). Compassionate mind training for people with high shame and self-criticism: Overview and pilot study of a group therapy approach. *Clinical Psychology & Psychotherapy*, 13(6),353–79. doi:10.1002/cpp.507

Goddard, E., Wingrove, J. & Moran, P. (2015). The impact of comorbid personality difficulties on response to IAPT treatment for depression and anxiety. *Behaviour Research and Therapy*, 73, 1–7. doi:10.1016/j.brat.2015.07.006

Gomez, R. & Corr, P. J. (2014). ADHD and personality: A meta-analytic review. *Clinical Psychology Review*, 34(5),376–88. doi:10.1016/j.cpr.2014.05.002

Gordon, R. M., Spektor, V. & Luu, L. (2019). Personality organization traits and expected countertransference and treatment interventions. *International Journal of Psychology and Psychoanalysis*, 5(1),1–7. doi:10.23937/2572-4037.1510039

Graham, E. K., Rutsohn, J. P., Turiano, N. A., et al. (2017). Personality predicts mortality risk: An integrative data analysis of 15 international longitudinal studies. *Journal of Research in Personality*, 70, 174–86. doi:10.1016/j.jrp.2017.07.005

Grant, B. F., Hasin, D. S., Stinson, F. S., et al. (2004). Prevalence, correlates, and disability of personality disorders in the United States: Results from the national epidemiologic survey on alcohol and related conditions. *Journal of Clinical Psychiatry*, 65(7),948–58. doi:10.4088/jcp.v65n0711

Griggs, S. M. & Tyrer, P. J. (1981). Personality disorder, social adjustment and treatment outcome in alcoholics. *Journal of Studies on Alcohol*, 42(9),802–5. doi:10.15288/jsa.1981.42.802

Grinker, R. R., Werble, B. & Drye, R. C. (1968). *The Borderline Syndrome: A Behavioral Study of Ego-Functions*, New York, Basic Books.

Grounds, A. & Gordon, H. (2007). In conversation with John Gunn. *Psychiatric Bulletin*, 31(1),25–8. doi:10.1192/pb.31.1.25

Gunderson, J., Masland, S. & Choi-Kain, L. (2018). Good psychiatric management: A review. *Current Opinion in Psychology*, 21, 127–31. doi:10.1016/j.copsyc.2017.12.006

Gunderson, J. G. & Lyons-Ruth, K. (2008). BPD's interpersonal hypersensitivity phenotype: A gene-environment-developmental model. *Journal of Personality Disorders*, 22(1),22–41. doi:10.1521/pedi.2008.22.1.22

Gunderson, J. G. & Singer, M. T. (1975). Defining borderline patients: An overview. *American Journal of Psychiatry*, 132(1),1–10. doi:10.1176/ajp.132.1.1

Gunderson, J. G., Stout, R. L., Mcglashan, T. H., et al. (2011). Ten-year course of borderline personality disorder: Psychopathology and function from the Collaborative Longitudinal Personality Disorders study.

Archives of General Psychiatry, 68(8),827–37. doi:10.1001/archgenpsychiatry.2011.37

Gunderson, J. G. & Zanarini, M. C. (2011). Deceptively simple – or radical shift? [Commentary]. *Personality and Mental Health*, 5(4),260–2. doi:10.1002/pmh.181

Gurven, M., Von Rueden, C., Massenkoff, M., Kaplan, H. & Lero Vie, M. (2013). How universal is the Big Five? Testing the five-factor model of personality variation among forager-farmers in the Bolivian Amazon. *Journal of Personality and Social Psychology*, 104(2),354–70. doi:10.1037/a0030841

Gutiérrez, F., Aluja, A., Peri, J. M., et al. (2015). Psychometric properties of the Spanish PID-5 in a clinical and a community sample. *Assessment*, 24(3),326–36. doi:10.1177/1073191115606518

Gutiérrez, F., Ruiz, J., Peri, J. M., Gárriz, M., Vall, G. & Cavero, M. (2019). Toward an integrated model of pathological personality traits: Common hierarchical structure of the PID-5 and the DAPP-BQ. *Journal of Personality Disorders*, 1-S18. doi:10.1521/pedi_2019_33_431

Haigh, R. & Pearce, S. (2017). *The Theory and Practice of Democratic Therapeutic Community Treatment*, London, Jessica Kingsley Publishers.

Hall, K., Barnicot, K., Crawford, M. & Moran, P. (2019). A systematic review of interventions aimed at improving the cardiovascular health of people diagnosed with personality disorders. *Social Psychiatry and Psychiatric Epidemiology*, 54(8),897–904. doi:10.1007/s00127-019-01705-x

Hansen, S. J., Christensen, S., Kongerslev, M. T., et al. (2019). Mental health professionals' perceived clinical utility of the ICD-10 vs. ICD-11 classification of personality disorders. *Personality and Mental Health*, 13 (2),84–95. doi:doi.org/10.1002/pmh.1442

Hare, R. D. (2003). *The Psychopathy Checklist – Revised* (2nd ed.), Toronto, Multi-Health Systems.

Harkness, A. R. & McNulty, J. L. (2006). An overview of personality: The MMPI-2 Personality Psychopathology Five (PSY-5) Scales. In Butcher, J. N. (ed.) *MMPI-2:*

A Practitioner's Guide. Washington, DC, American Psychological Association.

Hayes, S. C. (2004). Acceptance and Commitment Therapy and the new behavior therapies: Mindfulness, acceptance, and relationship. In Hayes, S. C., Follette, V. M. & Linehan, M. M. (eds.) *Mindfulness and Acceptance: Expanding the Cognitive-Behavioral Tradition*. New York, Guilford Press.

Hayes, S. C., Luoma, J. B., Bond, F. W., Masuda, A. & Lillis, J. (2006). Acceptance and Commitment Therapy: Model, processes and outcomes. *Behaviour Research and Therapy*, 44(1),1–25. doi:10.1016/j.brat.2005.06.006

Henderson, D. K. (1939). *Psychopathic States*, New York, W. W. Norton.

Henderson, D. K. & Gillespie, R. D. (1927). *A Text-Book of Psychiatry for Students and Practitioners* (1st ed.), Oxford, Oxford University Press.

Henry, D., Geary, D. & Tyrer, P. (1993). Adolf Hitler: A re-assessment of his personality status. *Irish Journal of Psychological Medicine*, 10(3),148–51. doi:10.1017/S0790966700012593

Herpertz, S. C., Huprich, S. K., Bohus, M., et al. (2017). The challenge of transforming the diagnostic system of personality disorders. *Journal of Personality Disorders*, 31(5),577–89. doi:10.1521/pedi_2017_31_338

Herpertz, S. C., Zanarini, M., Schulz, C. S., et al. (2007). World Federation of Societies of Biological Psychiatry (WFSBP) Guidelines for biological treatment of personality disorders. *World Journal of Biological Psychiatry*, 8(4),212–44. doi:10.1080/15622970701685224

Hershberger, A. R., Um, M. & Cyders, M. A. (2017). The relationship between the UPPS-P impulsive personality traits and substance use psychotherapy outcomes: A meta-analysis. *Drug and Alcohol Dependence*, 178, 408–16. doi:10.1016/j.drugalcdep.2017.05.032

Hoffmann, D., Rask, C. U., Hedman-Lagerlöf, E., Jensen, J. S. & Frostholm, L. (2020). Efficacy of internet-delivered Acceptance and Commitment Therapy for severe health anxiety: Results from a randomized, controlled trial. *Psychological Medicine*, 1–11. doi:10.1017/S0033291720001312

Hofmann, S. G., Anu Asnaani, M. A. & Hinton, D. E. (2010). Cultural aspects in social anxiety and social anxiety disorder. *Depression and Anxiety*, 27(12),1117–27. doi:10.1002/da.20759

Hopwood, C. J., Kotov, R., Krueger, R. F., et al. (2018). The time has come for dimensional personality disorder diagnosis. *Personality and Mental Health*, 12(1),82–6. doi:10.1002/pmh.1408

Hopwood, C. J., Morey, L. C., Donnellan, M. B., et al. (2013). Ten-year rank-order stability of personality traits and disorders in a clinical sample. *Journal of Personality*, 81(3),335–44. doi:10.1111/j.1467-6494.2012.00801.x

House, A. (15 September 2019a). Geoffrey Boycott and domestic abuse: A footnote on the psychiatric "evidence". Available from: https://profallanhouse.co.uk/geoffrey-boycott-and-domestic-abuse/ [Accessed 21 January 2021].

House, A. (2019b). *Understanding and Responding to Self-Harm: The One-Stop Guide: Practical Advice for Anybody Affected by Self-Harm*, London, Profile Books.

Høye, A., Jacobsen, B. K. & Hansen, V. (2013). Sex differences in mortality of admitted patients with personality disorders in North Norway: A prospective register study. *BMC Psychiatry*, 13, 317. doi:10.1186/1471-244X-13-317

Huang, Y., Kotov, R., De Girolamo, G., et al. (2009). DSM-IV personality disorders in the WHO World Mental Health Surveys. *British Journal of Psychiatry*, 195(1),46–53. doi:10.1192/bjp.bp.108.058552

Huband, N., McMurran, M., Evans, C. & Duggan, C. (2007). Social problem-solving plus psychoeducation for adults with personality disorder: Pragmatic randomised controlled trial. *British Journal of Psychiatry*, 190(4),307–13. doi:10.1192/bjp.bp.106.023341

Hunt, C. & Andrews, G. (1992). Measuring personality disorder: The use of self-report questionnaires. *Journal of Personality Disorders*, 6(2),125–33. doi:10.1521/pedi.1992.6.2.125

Huxley, E., Lewis, K. L., Coates, A. D., et al (2019). Evaluation of a brief intervention within a stepped care whole of service model for personality disorder. *BMC Psychiatry*, 19, 341. doi:10.1186/s12888-019-2308-z

Jackson, H. J. & Burgess, P. M. (2004). Personality disorders in the community: Results from the Australian National Survey of Mental Health and Well-Being Part III. *Social Psychiatry and Psychiatric Epidemiology*, 39(10)765–76. doi:10.1007/s00127-004-0821-x

James, W. (1890). *The Principles of Psychology*, New York, Henry Holt.

Jane, J. S., Oltmanns, T. F., South, S. C. & Turkheimer, E. (2007). Gender bias in diagnostic criteria for personality disorders: An item response theory analysis. *Journal of Abnormal Psychology*, 116(1),166–75. doi:10.1037/0021-843X.116.1.166

Jilek-Aall, L. (1988). Suicidal behaviour among youth: A cross-cultural comparison. *Transcultural Psychiatric Research Review*, 25 (2),87–105. doi:10.1177%2F136346158802500201

Johnson, F. (1985). The Western concept of self. In Marsella, A. J., De Vos, G. A. & Hsu, F. L. K. (eds.) *Culture and Self: Asian and Western Perspectives*. London, Tavistock.

Johnson, T. (1998). Clinical trials in psychiatry: Background and statistical perspective. *Statistical Methods in Medical Research*, 7 (3),209–34. doi:10.1177/096228029800700302

Jokela, M., Batty, G. D., Nyberg, S. T., et al. (2013). Personality and all-cause mortality: Individual-participant meta-analysis of 3,947 deaths in 76,150 adults. *American Journal of Epidemiology*, 178(5),667–75. doi:10.1093/aje/kwt170

Jones, M. (1968). *Beyond the Therapeutic Community: Social Learning and Social Psychiatry*, New Haven, CT, Yale University Press.

Jowett, S., Karatzias, T., Shevlin, M. & Albert, I. (2020). Differentiating symptom profiles of ICD-11 PTSD, complex PTSD, and borderline personality disorder: A latent class analysis in a multiply traumatized sample. *Personality Disorders: Theory, Research, and*

Treatment, 11(1),36–45. doi:10.1037/
per0000346

Kaess, M., Brunner, R. & Chanen, A. (2014).
Borderline personality disorder in
adolescence. *Pediatrics*, 134(4),782–93.
doi:10.1542/peds.2013-3677

Karukivi, M., Vahlberg, T., Horjamo, K.,
Nevalainen, M. & Korkeila, J. (2017). Clinical
importance of personality difficulties:
Diagnostically sub-threshold personality
disorders. *BMC Psychiatry*, 17(1),16.
doi:10.1186/s12888-017-1200-y

Kendall, T., Burbeck, R. & Bateman, A. (2010).
Pharmacotherapy for borderline personality
disorder: NICE guideline. *British Journal of
Psychiatry*, 196(2),158–9. doi:10.1192/
bjp.196.2.158

Kendell, R. E. (1991). The major functional
psychoses: Are they independent entities or
part of a continuum? Philosophical and
conceptual issues underlying the debate. In
Kerr, A. & Mcclelland, H. (eds.) *Concepts of
Mental Disorder: A Continuing Debate*.
London, Gaskell/Royal College of
Psychiatrists.

Kendell, R. E. (2002). The distinction between
personality disorder and mental illness.
British Journal of Psychiatry, 180(2),110–15.
doi:10.1192/bjp.180.2.110

Kendler, K. S., Neale, M. C., Kessler, R. C.,
Heath, A. C. & Eaves, L. J. (1993).
A longitudinal twin study of personality and
major depression in women. *Archives of
General Psychiatry*, 50(11),853–62.
doi:10.1001/archpsyc.1993.01820230023002

Kerber, A., Schultze, M., MüLler, S., et al. (2020).
Development of a short and ICD-11
compatible measure for DSM-5 maladaptive
personality traits using ant colony
optimization algorithms. *Psychological
Assessment*, doi:10.31234/osf.io/rsw54

Kernberg, O. (1967). Borderline personality
organization. *Journal of the American
Psychoanalytic Association*, 15(3),641–85.
doi:10.1177/000306516701500309

Kessler, R. C., Mcgonagle, K. A., Zhao, S., et al.
(1994). Lifetime and 12-month prevalence of
DSM-III-R psychiatric disorders in the
United States. Results from the National
Comorbidity Survey. *Archives of General*

Psychiatry, 51(1),8–19. doi:10.1001/
archpsyc.1994.03950010008002

Khalifa, N., Duggan, C., Stoffers, J., et al. (2010).
Pharmacological interventions for antisocial
personality disorder. *Cochrane Database of
Systematic Reviews*, (8), CD007667.
doi:10.1002/14651858.CD007667.pub2

Kim, J. J., Rapee, R. M., Oh, K. J. & Moon, H.-S.
(2008). Retrospective report of social
withdrawal during adolescence and current
maladjustment in young adulthood:
Cross-cultural comparisons between
Australian and South Korean students.
Journal of Adolescence, 31(5),543–63.
doi:10.1016/j.adolescence.2007.10.011

Kim, Y. R., Tyrer, P. & Hwang, S. T. (2021).
Personality Assessment Questionnaire for
ICD-11 personality trait domains:
Development and testing. *Personality and
Mental Health*, 10,58–71. doi:10.1002/
pmh.1493

Kim, Y. R., Tyrer, P., Lee, H.-S., et al. (2015).
Preliminary field trial of a putative research
algorithm for diagnosing ICD-11 personality
disorders in psychiatric patients: 2. Proposed
trait domains. *Personality and Mental Health*,
9(4),298–307. doi:10.1002/pmh.1305

Knight, R. P. (1953). Borderline states. *Bulletin
of the Menninger Clinic*, 17,1–12.

Köck, P. & Walter, M. (2018). Personality
disorder and substance use disorder – An
update. *Mental Health & Prevention*, 12,
82–9. doi:10.1016/j.mhp.2018.10.003

Koehler, J. A., Lösel, F., Akoensi, T. D. &
Humphreys, D. K. (2013). A systematic
review and meta-analysis on the effects of
young offender treatment programs in
Europe. *Journal of Experimental Criminology*,
9(1),19–43. doi:10.1007/s11292-012-9159-7

Koelen, J. A., Luyten, P., Eurelings-Bontekoe,
L. H. M., et al. (2012). The impact of level of
personality organization on treatment
response: A systematic review. *Psychiatry and
Clincal Neuroscience*, 75(4),355–74.
doi:10.1521/psyc.2012.75.4.355

Koenigsberg, H. W., Kernberg, O. F. &
Schomer, J. (1983). Diagnosing borderline
conditions in an outpatient setting. *Archives
of General Psychiatry*, 40(1),49–53.
doi:10.1001/archpsyc.1983.01790010051005

Kool, S., Dekker, J., Duijsens, I. J., De Jonghe, F. & Puite, B. (2003). Changes in personality pathology after pharmacotherapy and combined therapy for depressed patients. *Journal of Personality Disorders*, 17(1),60–72. doi:10.1521/pedi.17.1.60.24058

Kotov, R., Krueger, R. F., Watson, D., et al. (2021). The Hierarchical Taxonomy of Psychopathology (HiTOP): A quantitative nosology based on consensus of evidence. *Annual Review of Clinical Psychology*, 17, 83–108. doi:10.1146/annurev-clinpsy -081219-093304

Kraepelin, E. (1909–15). *Psychiatrie: Ein Lehrbuch für Studirende und Aerzte* (8th ed.), Leipzig, Barth.

Krasnova, A., Eaton, W. W. & Samuels, J. F. (2019). Antisocial personality and risks of cause-specific mortality: Results from the Epidemiologic Catchment Area study with 27 years of follow-up. *Social Psychiatry and Psychiatric Epidemiology*, 54(5),617–25. doi:10.1007/s00127-018-1628-5

Kretschmer, E. (1922) *Körperbau und Charakter.* Berlin, Springer.

Kroll, J., Sines, L., Martin, K., Lari, S., ., Pyle, R. & Zander, J. (1981). Borderline personality disorder: Construct validity of the concept. *Archives of General Psychiatry*, 38(9),1021–6. doi:10.1001/archpsyc.1981.01780340073009

Kulkarni, J. (2017). Complex PTSD – a better description for borderline personality disorder? *Australasian Psychiatry*, 25(4),333–5. doi:10.1177/1039856217700284

Laporte, L., Paris, J., Bergevin, T., Fraser, R. & Cardin, J. F. (2018). Clinical outcomes of a stepped care program for borderline personality disorder. *Personality and Mental Health*, 12(3),252–64. doi:10.1002/pmh.1421

Laurenssen, E., Luyten, P., Kikkert, M. J., et al. (2018). Day hospital mentalization-based treatment v. specialist treatment as usual in patients with borderline personality disorder: Randomized controlled trial. *Psychological Medicine*, 48(15),2522–9. doi:10.1017/S0033291718000132

Lee, C. K., Kwak, Y. S., Rhee, H., et al. (1987). The nationwide epidemiological study of mental disorders in Korea. *Journal of Korean Medical Science*, 2(1),19–34. doi:10.3346/jkms.1987.2.1.19

Lee, S. H. & Oh, K. S. (1999). Offensive type of social phobia: Cross-cultural perspectives. *International Medical Journal*, 6(4),271–80.

Lejuez, C. W. & Gratz, K. L. (eds.) (2020). *The Cambridge Handbook of Personality Disorders*, Cambridge, Cambridge University Press.

Lejuez, C. W., Hopko, D. R., Acierno, R., Daughters, S. B. & Pagoto, S. L. (2011). Ten year revision of the brief behavioral activation treatment for depression: Revised treatment manual. *Behavior Modification*, 35 (2),111–61. doi:10.1177/0145445510390929

Lester, R., Prescott, L., Mccormack, M., Sampson, M. & North West Boroughs Healthcare NHS Foundation Trust (2020). Service users' experiences of receiving a diagnosis of borderline personality disorder: A systematic review. *Personality and Mental Health*, 14 (3),263–83. doi:10.1002/pmh.1478

Levy, K. N., Mcmain, S., Bateman, A. & Clouthier, T. (2018). Treatment of borderline personality disorder. *Psychiatric Clinics of North America*, 41(4),711–28. doi:10.1016/j.psc.2018.07.011

Lewis, G. & Appleby, L. (1988). Personality disorder: The patients psychiatrists dislike. *British Journal of Psychiatry*, 153, 44–9. doi:10.1192/bjp.153.1.44

Li, J.-B., Vazsonyi, A. T. & Dou, K. (2018). Is individualism-collectivism associated with self-control? Evidence from Chinese and US samples. *PLOS One*, 13(12), e0208541. doi:10.1371/journal.pone.0208541

Lieb, K., Völlm, B., Rücker, G., Timmer, A. & Stoffers, J. M. (2010). Pharmacotherapy for borderline personality disorder: Cochrane systematic review of randomised trials. *British Journal of Psychiatry*, 196(1),4–12. doi:10.1192/bjp.bp.108.062984

Lier, H. Ø., Biringer, E., Stubhaug, B., Eriksen, H. R. & Tangen, T. (2011). Psychiatric disorders and participation in pre- and postoperative counselling groups in bariatric surgery patients. *Obesity Surgery*, 21 (6),730–7. doi:10.1007/s11695-010-0146-7

Linehan, M. M. (1987a). Dialectical behavior therapy for borderline personality disorder. Theory and method. *Bulletin of the Menninger Clinic*, 51(3),261–76.

Linehan, M. M. (1987b). Dialectical behavioral therapy: A cognitive behavioral approach to parasuicide. *Journal of Personality Disorders*, 1(4),328–33.

Linehan, M. M. (1993). *Cognitive Behaviural Treatment of Borderline Personality Disorder*, New York, Guilford Press.

Linehan, M. M. (2019). *How Marsha Linehan Developed the Central Feature of Dialectical Behavior Therapy. A descent into despair led to the birth of dialectical behavior therapy* [Online]. Psychology Today. Available: https://www.psychologytoday.com/nz/articles/201912/how-marsha-linehan-developed-the-central-feature-dialectical-behavior-therapy [Accessed 10 February 2021].

Linehan, M. M., Armstrong, H. E., Suarez, A., Allmon, D. & Heard, H. L. (1991). Cognitive-behavioral treatment of chronically parasuicidal borderline patients. *Archives of General Psychiatry*, 48(12),1060–4. doi:10.1001/archpsyc.1991.01810360024003

Linehan, M. M. & Dexter-Mazza, E. T. (2008). Dialectical behavior therapy for borderline personality disorder. In Barlow, D. H. (ed.) *Clinical Handbook of Psychological Disorders: A Step-by-Step Treatment Manual*. 4th ed. New York, Guilford Press.

Linehan, M. M., Dimeff, L. A., Reynolds, S. K., et al. (2002). Dialectical behavior therapy versus comprehensive validation therapy plus 12-step for the treatment of opioid dependent women meeting criteria for borderline personality disorder. *Drug and Alcohol Dependence*, 67(1),13–26. doi:10.1016/s0376-8716(02)00011-x

Livesley, W. J. (2003). *Practical Management of Personality Disorder*, New York, Guilford Press.

Livesley, W. J. (2021). Why is an evidence-based classification of personality disorder so elusive? *Personality and Mental Health*, 15 (1),8–25. doi:10.1002/pmh.1471

Livesley, W. J. & Larstone, R. (eds.) (2018). *Handbook of Personality Disorders: Theory, Research, and Treatment*, (2nd), New York, Guilford Press.

Livesley, W. J., Schroeder, M. L., Jackson, D. N. & Jang, K. L. (1994). Categorical distinctions in the study of personality disorder: Implications for classification. *Journal of Abnormal Psychology*, 103(1),6–17. doi:10.1037//0021-843x.103.1.6

Löckenhoff, C. E., Chan, W., McCrae, R. R., et al. (2014). Gender stereotypes of personality: Universal and accurate? *Journal of Cross-Cultural Psychology*, 45(5),675–94. doi:10.1177/0022022113520075

Loranger, A. W. (1999). *The International Personality Disorder Examination (IPDE)*, Odessa, FL, Psychological Assessment Resources.

Loranger, A. W., Sartorius, N., Andreoli, A., et al. (1994). The International Personality Disorder Examination. The World Health Organization/Alcohol, Drug Abuse, and Mental Health Administration international pilot study of personality disorders. *Archives of General Psychiatry*, 51(3),215–24. doi:10.1001/archpsyc.1994.03950030051005

Lotfi, M., Bach, B., Amini, M. & Simonsen, E. (2018). Structure of DSM-5 and ICD-11 personality domains in Iranian community sample. *Personality and Mental Health*, 12(2),155–69. doi:10.1002/pmh.1409

Lynch, T. R., Hempel, R. J. & Dunkley, C. (2015). Radically open-dialectical behavior therapy for disorders of over-control: Signaling matters. *American Journal of Psychotherapy*, 69(2),141–62. doi:10.1176/appi.psychotherapy.2015.69.2.141

Macdonald, K. (1998). Evolution, culture, and the five-factor model. *Journal of Cross-Cultural Psychology*, 29(1),119–49. doi:10.1177%2F0022022198291007

Mack, J. E. (1975). Borderline states: An historical perspective. In Mack, J. E. (ed.) *Borderline States in Psychiatry*. New York, Grune & Stratton Inc.

Main, T. F. (1946). The hospital as a therapeutic institution. *Bulletin of the Menninger Clinic*, 10, 66–70.

Makris, N., Oscar-Berman, M., Jaffin, S. K., et al. (2008). Decreased volume of the brain reward system in alcoholism. *Biological Psychiatry*, 64(3),192–202. doi:10.1016/j.biopsych.2008.01.018

Mannuzza, S., Klein, R. G., Bonagura, N., Malloy, P., Giampino, T. L. & Addalli, K. A. (1991). Hyperactive boys almost grown up: V. Replication of psychiatric status. *Archives of General Psychiatry*, 48(1),77–83. doi:10.1001/archpsyc.1991.01810250079012

Markon, K. E., Krueger, R. F. & Watson, D. (2005). Delineating the structure of normal and abnormal personality: An integrative hierarchical approach. *Journal of Personality and Social Psychology*, 88(1),139–57. doi:10.1037/0022-3514.88.1.139

Markus, H. R. & Kitayama, S. (1991). Culture and the self: Implications for cognition, emotion and motivation. *Psychological Review*, 98(2),224–53. doi:10.1037/0033-295X.98.2.224

Martinussen, M., Friborg, O., Schmierer, P., et al. (2017). The comorbidity of personality disorders in eating disorders: A meta-analysis. *Eating and Weight Disorders – Studies on Anorexia, Bulimia and Obesity*, 22, 201–9. doi:10.1007/s40519-016-0345-x

Matthews, G., Deary, I. J. & Whiteman, M. C. (2009). *Personality Traits* (3rd ed.), Cambridge, Cambridge University Press.

Matthies, S. & Philipsen, A. (2016). Comorbidity of personality disorders and adult Attention Deficit Hyperactivity Disorder (ADHD) – Review of recent findings. *Current Psychiatry Reports*, 18(4),33. doi:10.1007/s11920-016-0675-4

Maudsley, H. (1868). *The Physiology and Pathology of Mind* (2nd ed.), London, Macmillan.

McCrae, R. R. & Costa, P. T., Jr. (1984). *Emerging Lives, Enduring Dispositions: Personality in Adulthood*, Boston, MA, Little, Brown and Co.

McCrae, R. R., Yik, M. S., Trapnell, P. D., Bond, M. H. & Paulhus, D. L. (1998). Interpreting personality profiles across cultures: Bilingual, acculturation, and peer rating studies of Chinese undergraduates. *Journal of Personality and Social Psychology*, 74(4),1041–55.

McGilloway, A., Hall, R. E., Lee, T. & Bhui, K. S. (2010). A systematic review of personality disorder, race and ethnicity: Prevalence, aetiology and treatment. *BMC Psychiatry*, 10, 33. doi:10.1186/1471-244X-10-33

McMurran, M. (2020). Outcomes. In Ramsden, J., Prince, S. & Blazdell, J. (eds.) *Working Effectively with 'Personality Disorder': Contemporary and Critical Approaches to Clinical and Organizational Practice*. London, Luminate (Pavilion Publishing and Media Ltd).

McMurran, M., Crawford, M. J., Reilly, J. G., et al. (2011). Psycho-education with problem solving (PEPS) therapy for adults with personality disorder: A pragmatic multi-site community-based randomised clinical trial. *Trials*, 12, 198. doi:10.1186/1745-6215-12-198

McMurran, M., Crawford, M. J., Reilly, J., et al. (2016). Psychoeducation with problem-solving (PEPS) therapy for adults with personality disorder: A pragmatic randomised controlled trial to determine the clinical effectiveness and cost-effectiveness of a manualised intervention to improve social functioning. *Health Technology Assessment*, 20(52),1–250. doi:10.3310/hta20520

McMurran, M., Day, F., Reilly, J., et al. (2017). Psychoeducation and problem solving (PEPS) therapy for adults with personality disorder: A pragmatic randomized-controlled trial. *Journal of Personality Disorders*, 31(6),810–26. doi:10.1521/pedi_2017_31_286

Meyer, A. (1950). *The Collected Papers of Adolf Meyer*, Balitmore, MD, Johns Hopkins Press.

Miller, T. Q., Smith, T. W., Turner, C. W., Guijarro, M. L. & Hallet, A. J. (1996). A meta-analytic review of research on hostility and physical health. *Psychological Bulletin*, 119(2),322–48. doi:10.1037/0033-2909.119.2.322

Miller, T. W. & Kraus, R. F. (2007). Modified dialectical behavior therapy and problem solving for obsessive-compulsive personality disorder. *Journal of Contemporary Psychotherapy*, 37(2),79–85. doi:10.1007/s10879-006-9039-4

Millon, T. (1987). On the genesis and prevalence of borderline personality disorders: A social learning thesis. *Journal of Personality Disorders*, 1(4),354–72. doi:10.1521/pedi.1987.1.4.354

Mills, J. & Clark, M. S. (1982). Exchange and communal relationships. In Wheeler, L. (ed.) *Review of Personality and Social Psychology*. Beverly Hills, CA, Sage.

MIND. (2018). 'Shining lights in dark corners of people's lives' The Consensus Statement for People with Complex Mental Health Difficulties who are diagnosed with a Personality Disorder. Available: www.mind.org.uk/media-a/4408/consensus-statement-final.pdf.

MIND. (2020). *Personality disorders* [Online]. MIND. Available: www.mind.Org.Uk/Information-Support/Types-Of-Mental-Health-Problems/Personality-Disorders/Why-Is-It-Controversial/ [Accessed November 18 2020].

Minkov, M., Dutt, P., Schachner, M., et al. (2017). A revision of Hofstede's individualism-collectivism dimension A new national index from a 56-country study. *Cross Cultural & Strategic Management*, 24(3),386–404. doi:10.1108/CCSM-11-2016-0197

Moos, R. H. & Solomon, G. F. (1965). Psychologic comparisons between women with rheumatoid arthritis and their nonarthritic sisters. I. Personality test and interview rating data. *Psychosomatic Medicine*, 27, 135–49. doi:10.1097/00006842-196503000-00006

Moran, P., Leese, M., Lee, T., Walters, P., Thornicroft, G. & Mann, A. (2003). Standardised Assessment of Personality – Abbreviated Scale (SAPAS): Preliminary validation of a brief screen for personality disorder. *British Journal of Psychiatry*, 183 (3),228–32. doi:10.1192/bjp.183.3.228

Moran, P., Rendu, A., Jenkins, R., Tylee, A. & Mann, A. (2001). The impact of personality disorder in UK primary care: A 1-year follow-up of attenders. *Psychological Medicine*, 31(8),1447–54. doi:10.1017/s003329170105450z

Moran, P., Stewart, R., Brugha, T., et al. (2007). Personality disorder and cardiovascular disease: Results from a national household survey. *Journal of Clinical Psychiatry*, 68 (1),69–74. doi:10.4088/jcp.v68n0109

Mordekar, A. & Spence, S. (2008). Personality disorder in older people: How common is it and what can be done? *Advances in Psychiatric Treatment*, 14(1),71–7. doi:10.1192/apt.bp.107.003897

Morel, B. A. (1852). *Études cliniques: Traité, théorique et pratique des maladies mentales*, Nancy, Grimblot.

Morey, L. C., Berghuis, H., Bender, D. S., Verheul, R., Krueger, R. F. & Skodol, A. E. (2011). Toward a model for assessing level of personality functioning in DSM-5, Part II: Empirical articulation of a core dimension of personality pathology. *Journal of Personality Assessment*, 93(4),347–53. doi:10.1080/00223891.2011.577853

Morey, L. C., Krueger, R. F. & Skodol, A. E. (2013). The hierarchical structure of clinician ratings of proposed DSM-5 pathological personality traits. *Journal of Abnormal Psychology*, 122 (3),836–41. doi:10.1037/a0034003

Morey, L. C., Shea, M. T., Markowitz, J. C., et al. (2010). State effects of major depression on the assessment of personality and personality disorder. *American Journal of Psychiatry*, 167 (5),528–35. doi:10.1176/appi.ajp.2009.09071023

Morton, J., Snowdon, S., Gopold, M. & Guymer, E. (2012). Acceptance and Commitment Therapy group treatment for symptoms of borderline personality disorder: A public sector pilot study. *Cognitive and Behavioral Practice*, 19(4),527–44. doi:10.1016/j.cbpra.2012.03.005

Mulder, R. T. (1992). Boundaries of psychiatry. *Perspectives in Biology and Medicine*, 35 (3),443–59. doi:10.1353/pbm.1992.0027

Mulder, R. T. (2002). Personality pathology and treatment outcome in major depression: A review. *American Journal of Psychiatry*, 159 (3),359–71. doi:10.1176/appi.ajp.159.3.359

Mulder, R. T. (2004). Depression and personality disorder. In Joyce, P. R. & Mitchell, P. B. (eds.) *Mood Disorders: Recognition and Treatment*. Sydney, The University of New South Wales Press Ltd.

Mulder, R. T. (2008). An epidemic of depression or the medicalization of distress? *Perspectives in Biology and Medicine*, 51(2),238–50. doi:10.1353/pbm.0.0009

Mulder, R. T., Horwood, L. J. & Tyrer, P. (2020). The borderline pattern descriptor in the International Classification of Diseases, 11th Revision: A redundant addition to classification. *Australian & New Zealand Journal of Psychiatry*, 54(11),1095–100. doi:10.1177/0004867420951608

Mulder, R. T., Horwood, J., Tyrer, P., Carter, J. & Joyce, P. R. (2016). Validating the proposed ICD-11 domains. *Personality and Mental Health*, 10(2),84–95. doi:10.1002/pmh.1336

Mulder, R. T., Joyce, P. R. & Luty, S. E. (2003). The relationship of personality disorders to treatment outcome in depressed outpatients. *Journal of Clinical Psychiatry*, 64(3),259–64. doi:10.4088/jcp.v64n0306

Mulder, R. T., Murray, G. & Rucklidge, J. (2017). Common versus specific factors in psychotherapy: Opening the black box. *Lancet Psychiatry*, 4(12),953–62. doi:10.1016/S2215-0366(17)30100-1

Mulder, R. T., Newton-Howes, G., Crawford, M. J. & Tyrer, P. J. (2011). The central domains of personality pathology in psychiatric patients. *Journal of Personality Disorders*, 25(3),364–77. doi:10.1521/pedi.2011.25.3.364

Mulder, R. T. & Tyrer, P. (2019). Diagnosis and classification of personality disorders: Novel approaches. *Current Opinion in Psychiatry*, 32(1),27–31. doi:10.1097/YCO.0000000000000461

Mullins-Sweatt, S. N., Hopwood, C. J., Chmielewski, M., et al. (2020). Treatment of personality pathology through the lens of the hierarchical taxonomy of psychopathology: Developing a research agenda. *Personality and Mental Health*, 14(1),123–41. doi:10.1002/pmh.1464

Munjiza, J., Britvic, D. & Crawford, M. J. (2019). Lasting personality pathology following exposure to severe trauma in adulthood: Retrospective cohort study. *BMC Psychiatry*, 19(1),3. doi:10.1186/s12888-018-1975-5

Murphy, J. M. (1976). Psychiatric labeling in cross-cultural perspective. *Science*, 191 (4231),1019–28. doi:10.1126/science.1251213

Nandi, D. N., Banerjee, G., Nandi, S. & Nandi, P. (1992). Is hysteria on the wane? A community survey in West Bengal, India *British Journal of Psychiatry*, 160(1),87–91 doi:10.1192/bjp.160.1.87

National Health and Medical Research Council (2012). *Clinical Practice Guideline for the Management of Borderline Personality Disorder*, Melbourne, National Health and Medical Research Council.

National Institute for Health and Care Excellence (2009). *Borderline Personality Disorder: Recognition and Management (NICE Clinical Guideline CG78)*. London, NICE.

National Institute for Health and Care Excellence (2009; updated 2013). *Antisocial Personality Disorder: Prevention and Management (NICE Clinical guideline CG77)*. London, NICE.

Neacsiu, A. D., Erberle, J. W., Keng, S.-L., Fang, C. M. & Rosenthal, M. Z. (2017). Understanding borderline personality disorder across sociocultural groups: Findings, issues, and future directions. *Current Psychiatry Reviews*, 13(3),188–223. doi:10.2174/1573400513666170612122034

Newton-Howes, G., Clark, L. A. & Chanen, A. (2015a). Personality disorder across the life course. *Lancet*, 385(9969),727–34. doi:10.1016/S0140-6736(14)61283-6

Newton-Howes, G. & Foulds, J. (2018). Personality disorder and alcohol use disorder: An overview. *Psychopathology*, 51 (2),130–36. doi:10.1159/000486602

Newton-Howes, G. M., Foulds, J. A., Guy, N. H., Boden, J. M. & Mulder, R. T. (2017). Personality disorder and alcohol treatment outcome: Systematic review and meta-analysis. *British Journal of Psychiatry*, 211(1),22–30. doi:10.1192/bjp.bp.116.191720

Newton-Howes, G. & Mulder, R. T. (2020). Treatment and management of personality disorder. In Geddes, J. R., Andreasen, N. C. & Goodwin, G. M. (eds.) *New Oxford Textbook of Psychiatry*. 3rd ed. Oxford, Oxford University Press.

Newton-Howes, G., Mulder, R. T. & Tyrer, P. (2015b). Diagnostic neglect: The potential impact of losing a separate axis for personality disorder. *British Journal of Psychiatry*, 206(5),355–6. doi:10.1192/bjp.bp.114.155259

Newton-Howes, G., Tyrer, P., Anagnostakis, K., et al. (2010). The prevalence of personality disorder, its comorbidity with mental state disorders, and its clinical significance in community mental health teams. *Social Psychiatry and Psychiatric Epidemiology*, 45 (4),453–60. doi:10.1007/s00127-009-0084-7

Newton-Howes, G., Tyrer, P., Johnson, T., et al. (2014). Influence of personality on the outcome of treatment in depression: Systematic review and meta-analysis. *Journal of Personality Disorders*, 28(4),577–93. doi:10.1521/pedi_2013_27_070

Newton-Howes, G., Tyrer, P., North, B. & Yang, M. (2008a). The prevalence of personality disorder in schizophrenia and psychotic disorders: Systematic review of rates and explanatory modelling. *Psychological Medicine*, 38(8),1075–82. doi:10.1017/S0033291707002036

Newton-Howes, G., Weaver, T. & Tyrer, P. (2008b). Attitudes of staff towards patients with personality disorder in community mental health teams. *Australian & New Zealand Journal of Psychiatry*, 42(7),572–7. doi:10.1080/00048670802119739

Ni, H. C. & Gau, S. S. (2015). Co-occurrence of attention-deficit hyperactivity disorder symptoms with other psychopathology in young adults: Parenting style as a moderator. *Comprehensive Psychiatry*, 57, 85–96. doi:10.1016/j.comppsych.2014.11.002

Norasakkunkit, V. & Uchida, Y. (2014). To conform or to maintain self-consistency? Hikikomori risk in Japan and the deviation from seeking harmony. *Journal of Social and Clinical Psychology*, 33(10),918–35. doi:10.1521/jscp.2014.33.10.918

Nordentoft, M., Thorup, A., Petersen, L., et al. (2006). Transition rates from schizotypal disorder to psychotic disorder for first-contact patients included in the OPUS trial. A randomized clinical trial of integrated treatment and standard treatment. *Schizophrenia Research*, 83(1),29–40. doi:10.1016/j.schres.2006.01.002

O'Boyle, M. (1995). DSM-III-R and Eysenck personality measures among patients in a substance abuse programme. *Personality and Individual Differences*, 18(4),561–5.

O'Neil, A., Jacka, F. N., Quirk, S. E., et al. (2015). A shared framework for the common mental disorders and non-communicable disease: Key considerations for disease prevention and control. *BMC Psychiatry*, 15, 15. doi:10.1186/s12888-015-0394-0

Olabi, B. & Hall, J. (2010). Borderline personality disorder: Current drug treatments and future prospects. *Therapeutic Advances in Chronic Disease*, 1(2),59–66. doi:10.1177/2040622310368455

Olajide, K., Munjiza, J., Moran, P., et al. (2018). Development and psychometric properties of the Standardized Assessment of Severity of Personality Disorder (SASPD). *Journal of Personality Disorders*, 32(1),44–56. doi:10.1521/pedi_2017_31_285

Oltmanns, J. R. & Widiger, T. A. (2018). A self-report measure for the ICD-11 dimensional trait model proposal: The personality inventory for ICD-11. *Psychological Assessment*, 30(2),154–69. doi:10.1037/pas0000459

Oltmanns, J. R. & Widiger, T. A. (2019). Evaluating the assessment of the ICD-11 personality disorder diagnostic system. *Psychological Assessment*, 31(5),674–84. doi:10.1037/pas0000693

Oltmanns, J. R. & Widiger, T. A. (2020). The Five-Factor Personality Inventory for ICD-11: A facet-level assessment of the ICD-11 trait model. *Psychological Assessment*, 32(1),60–71. doi:10.1037/pas0000763

Oltmanns, T. F. & Balsis, S. (2011). Personality disorders in later life: Questions about the measurement, course, and impact of disorders. *Annual Review of Clinical Psychology*, 7, 321–49. doi:10.1146/annurev-clinpsy-090310-120435

Orwell, G. (1940). Charles Dickens. *Inside the Whale and Other Essays*. London, Victor Gollancz Ltd.

Oyserman, D., Coon, H. M. & Kemmelmeier, M. (2002). Rethinking individualism and collectivism: Evaluation of theoretical assumptions and meta-analyses. *Psychological Bulletin*, 128(1),3–72. doi:10.1037/0033-2909.128.1.3

Papamalis, F. E., Kalyva, E., Teare, M. D. & Meier, P. S. (2020). The role of personality functioning in drug misuse treatment engagement. *Addiction*, 115(4),726–39. doi:10.1111/add.14872

Paris, J. (1991). Personality disorders, parasuicide and culture. *Transcultural Psychiatric Research Review*, 28(1),25–39. doi:10.1177%2F136346159102800102

Paris, J. (1994). The etiology of borderline personality disorder: A biopsychosocial approach. *Psychiatry*, 57(4),316–25. doi:10.1080/00332747.1994.11024696

Paris, J. (1998). Personality disorders in sociocultural perspective. *Journal of Personality Disorders*, 12(4),289–301. doi:10.1521/pedi.1998.12.4.289

Paris, J. (2020). Access to psychotherapy for patients with personality disorders. *Personality and Mental Health*, 14(3),246–53. doi:10.1002/pmh.1483

Paris, J. & Lis, E. (2013). Can sociocultural and historical mechanisms influence the development of borderline personality disorder? *Transcultural Psychiatry*, 50 (1),140–51. doi:10.1177/1363461512468105

Parsonage, M., Hard, E. & Rock, B. (2014). *Managing Patients with Complex Needs: Evaluation of the City and Hackney Primary Care Psychotherapy Consultation Service*, London, Centre for Mental Health.

Pascual, J. C., Malagón, A., Córcoles, D., et al. (2008). Immigrants and borderline personality disorder at a psychiatric emergency service. *British Journal of Psychiatry*, 193(6),471–6. doi:10.1192/bjp. bp.107.038208

Paykel, E. S. (1972). Depressive typologies and response to amitriptyline. *British Journal of Psychiatry*, 120(555),147–56. doi:10.1192/ bjp.120.555.147

Peabody, F. W. (1927). The care of the patient. *JAMA*, 88(12),877–82. doi:10.1001/ jama.1927.02680380001001

Pearce, S. (2007). Knowledge of the effectiveness of treatments for borderline personality disorder is not yet sufficient to justify the lack of a control condition [Letter to the Editor]. *Archives of General Psychiatry*, 64(5),609. doi:10.1001/ archpsyc.64.5.609-b

Pearce, S. & Haigh, R. (2008). Mini therapeutic communities – A new development in the United Kingdom. *Therapeutic Communities*, 29(2),111–24.

Pearce, S., Scott, L., Attwood, G., Saunders, K., et al. (2017). Democratic therapeutic community treatment for personality disorder: Randomised controlled trial. *British Journal of Psychiatry*, 210(2),149–56. doi:10.1192/bjp.bp.116.184366

Pelizza, L. & Pupo, S. (2016). Brittle diabetes: Psychopathology and personality. *Journal of Diabetes and its Complications*, 30(8),1544–7. doi:10.1016/j.jdiacomp.2016.07.028

Peralta, V., Cuesta, M. J. & De Leon, J. (1991). Premorbid personality and positive and negative symptoms in schizophrenia. *Acta Psychiatrica Scandinavica*, 84(4),336–9. doi:10.1111/j.1600-0447.1991.tb03156.x

Perry, J. C. & Klerman, G. L. (1978). The borderline patient. A comparative analysis of four sets of diagnostic criteria. *Archives of General Psychiatry*, 35(2),141–50. doi:10.1001/archpsyc.1978.01770260019001

Petursson, H. & Lader, M. H. (1981). Withdrawal from long-term benzodiazepine treatment. *British Medical Journal (Clinical Research Ed.)*, 283(6292),643–5. doi:10.1136/ bmj.283.6292.643

Pfohl, B., Coryell, W., Zimmerman, M. & Stangl, D. (1986). DSM-III personality disorders: Diagnostic overlap and internal consistency of individual DSM-III criteria. *Comprehensive Psychiatry*, 27 (1),21–34. doi:10.1016/0010-440x(86) 90066-0

Pilgrim, D. (2018). Taming the Beast Within: Shredding the Stereotypes of Personality Disorder, by Peter Tyrer [Book Review]. Available: https://www.timeshighereducation .com/books/review-taming-the-beast-within- peter-tyrer-sheldon-press].

Pinel, P. (1809). *Traité médico-philosophique sur l'aliénation mentale* (2nd ed.), Paris, Chez J Ant Brosson.

Pope, H. G., Jonas, J. M., Hudson, J. I., Cohen, B. M. & Gunderson, J. G. (1983). The validity of DSM-III borderline personality disorder: A phenomenologic, family history, treatment response, and long-term follow-up study. *Archives of General Psychiatry*, 40 (1),23–30. doi:10.1001/archpsyc.1983.01790010025003

Preston, N. (2015). Psychologically Informed Planned Environments (PIPEs): Empowering the institutionalised prisoner. *Forensic Update*, (117),7–14.

Prichard, J. C. (1837). *A treatise on insanity and other diseases affecting the mind*, Philadelphia, PA, Haswell, Barrington, and Haswell.

Quirk, S. E., El-Gabalawy, R., Brennan, S. L., et al. (2015). Personality disorders and physical comorbidities in adults from the United States: Data from the National Epidemiologic Survey on Alcohol and Related Conditions. *Social Psychiatry and Psychiatric Epidemiology*, 50, 807–80. doi:10.1007/s00127-014-0974-1

Ramsden, J., Prince, S. & Blazdell, J. (eds.) (2020). *Working Effectively with 'Personality Disorder': Contemporary and Critical Approaches to Clinical and Organizational Practice*, London, Luminate (Pavilion Publishing and Media Ltd).

Ranger, M., Tyrer, P., Miloseska, K., et al. (2009). Cost-effectiveness of nidotherapy for comorbid personality disorder and severe mental illness: Randomized controlled trial. *Epidemiologia e Psichiatria Sociale*, 18 (2),128–36. doi:10.1017/S1121189X00001019

Rapoport, R. N. (1960). *Community as Doctor: New Perspectives on a Therapeutic Community*, London, Tavistock Publications.

Reich, J., Schatzberg, A. & Delucchi, K. (2018). Empirical evidence of the effect of personality pathology on the outcome of panic disorder. *Journal of Psychiatric Research*, 107, 42–7. doi:10.1016/j.jpsychires.2018.10.005

Ring, D. & Lawn, S. (2019). Stigma perpetuation at the interface of mental health care: A review to compare patient and clinician perspectives of stigma and borderline personality disorder. *Journal of Mental Health*, 1–21. doi:10.1080/09638237.2019.1581337

Roberts, B. W. & Delvecchio, W. F. (2000). The rank-order consistency of personality traits from childhood to old age: A quantitative review of longitudinal studies. *Psychological Bulletin*, 126(1),3–25. doi:10.1037/0033-2909.126.1.3

Roberts, B. W., Hill, P. L. & Davis, J. P. (2017a). How to change conscientiousness: The sociogenomic trait intervention model. *Personality Disorders: Theory, Research, and Treatment*, 8(3),199–205. doi:10.1037/per0000242

Roberts, B. W., Luo, J., Briley, D. A., Chow, P. I., Su, R. & Hill, P. L. (2017b). A systematic review of personality trait change through intervention. *Psychological Bulletin*, 143 (2),117–41. doi:10.1037/bul0000088

Roberts, B. W. & Robins, R. W. (2004). Person-Environment Fit and its implications for personality development: A longitudinal study. *Journal of Personality*, 72(1),89–110. doi:10.1111/j.0022-3506.2004.00257.x

Robin, A. (1976). Rationing out-patients: A defence of the waiting list. *British Journal of Psychiatry*, 129(2),138–41. doi:10.1192/bjp.129.2.138

Robins, L. N. (1966). *Deviant Children Grown Up: A Sociological and Psychiatric Study of Sociopathic Personality*, Baltimore, MD, Williams & Wilkins.

Ronningstam, E. (2010). Narcissistic personality disorder: A current review. *Current Psychiatry Reports*, 12(1),68–75. doi:10.1007/s11920-009-0084-z

Rosenström, T., Torvik, F. A., Ystrom, E., et al. (2018). Prediction of alcohol use disorder using personality disorder traits: A twin study. *Addiction*, 113(1),15–24. doi:10.1111/add.13951

Rossier, J. & Rigozzi, C. (2008). Personality disorders and the five-factor model among French speakers in Africa and Europe. *Canadian Journal of Psychiatry*, 53(8),534–44. doi:10.1177%2F070674370805300808

Royal College of Psychiatrists (2020). *Services for people diagnosable with personality disorder [Position Statement PS01/20]*. London, Royal College of Psychiatrists.

Rutter, M. & Smith, D. J. (eds.) (1995). *Psychosocial Disorders in Young People. Time Trends and Their Causes*, Chichester, John Wiley & Sons.

Ryle, A. (ed.) (1997). *Cognitive Analytic Therapy and Borderline Personality Disorder: The Model and the Method*, Chichester, Wiley.

Ryle, A. (2004). The contribution of cognitive analytic therapy to the treatment of borderline personality disorder. *Journal of Personality Disorders*, 18(1),3–35. doi:10.1521/pedi.18.1.3.32773

Ryle, A. & Kellett, S. (2018). Cognitive analytic therapy. In Livesley, W. J. & Larstone, R. (eds.) *Handbook of Personality Disorders: Theory, Research, and Treatment*. 2nd ed. New York, Guilford Press.

Sampath, H. M. (1974). Prevalence of psychiatric disorders in a Southern Baffin Island Eskimo Settlement. *Canadian Psychiatric Association Journal*, 19(4),363–7. doi:10.1177/070674377401900406

Samuels, J. (2011). Personality disorders: Epidemiology and public health issues. *International Review of Psychiatry*, 23 (3),223–33. doi:10.3109/09540261.2011.588200

Samuels, J., Eaton, W. W., Bienvenu, O. J., 3rd., Brown, C. H., Costa, P. T., Jr. & Nestadt, G. (2002). Prevalence and correlates of personality disorders in a community sample. *British Journal of Psychiatry*, 180 (6),536–42. doi:10.1192/bjp.180.6.536

Santayana, G. (1905). *Introduction and Reason in Common Sense (The Life of Reason: The Phases of Human Progress. Vol 1.)*, New York, Scribner.

Santos, H. C., Varnum, M. E. W. & Grossmann, I. (2017). Global increases in individualism. *Psychological Science*, 28 (9),1228–39. doi:10.1177/0956797617700622

Sartorius, N. & Schulze, H. (2005). *Reducing the Stigma of Mental Illness: A Report from a Global Programme of the World Psychiatric Association*, Cambridge, Cambridge University Press.

Sato, T. & Takeichi, M. (1993). Lifetime prevalence of specific psychiatric disorders in a general medicine clinic. *General Hospital Psychiatry*, 15(4),224–33. doi:10.1016/0163-8343(93)90037-O

Saucier, G. (2002). Orthogonal markers for orthogonal factors: The case of the Big Five. *Journal of Research in Personality*, 36(1),1–31. doi:10.1006/jrpe.2001.2335

Sauer-Zavala, S., Bentley, K. H. & Wilner, J. G. (2016). Transdiagnostic treatment of borderline personality disorder and comorbid disorders: A clinical replication series. *Journal of Personality Disorders*, 30 (1),35–51. doi:10.1521/pedi_2015_29_179

Schmideberg, M. (1947). The treatment of psychopaths and borderline patients. *American Journal of Psychotherapy*, 1 (1),45–70. doi:10.1176/appi.psychotherapy.1947.1.1.45

Schneider, K. (1921). *Studien über Persönlichkeit und Schicksal Eingeschriebener Prostituierter*, Berlin, Springer.

Schneider, K. (1923). *Die Psychopathischen Persönlichkeiten*, Leipzig & Wien, Franz Deuticke.

Schulz, S. C., Zanarini, M. C., Bateman, A., et al. (2008). Olanzapine for the treatment of borderline personality disorder: Variable dose 12-week randomised double-blind placebo-controlled study. *British Journal of Psychiatry*, 193(6),485–92. doi:10.1192/bjp.bp.107.037903

Schuster, J.-P., Hoertel, N., Le Strat, Y., Manetti, A. & Limosin, F. (2013). Personality disorders in older adults: Findings from the National Epidemiologic Survey on Alcohol and Related Conditions. *American Journal of Geriatric Psychiatry*, 21, 757–68. doi:10.1016/j.jagp.2013.01.055

Schweizer, E., Rickels, K., De Martinis, N., Case, G. & García-España, F. (1998). The effect of personality on withdrawal severity and taper outcome in benzodiazepine dependent patients. *Psychological Medicine*, 28(3),713–20. doi:10.1017/s0033291798006540

Seivewright, H., Tyrer, P. & Johnson, T. (2002). Change in personality status in neurotic disorders [Research Letter]. *Lancet*, 359 (9325),2253–4. doi:10.1016/S0140-6736(02)09266-8

Sellbom, M., Bach, B. & Huxley, E. (2018). Related personality disorders located within an elaborated externalizing psychopathology spectrum. In Lochman, J. E. & Matthys, W. (eds.) *The Wiley Handbook of Disruptive and Impulse-Control Disorders*. Chichester, John Wiley & Sons.

Sharp, C. (2016). Current trends in BPD research as indicative of a broader sea-change in psychiatric nosology. *Personality Disorders: Theory, Research, and Treatment*, 7 (4),334–43. doi:10.1037/per0000199

Sharp, C., Wright, A. G., Fowler, J. C., et al. (2015). The structure of personality pathology: Both general ('g') and specific ('s') factors? *Journal of Abnormal Psychology*, 124 (2),387–98. doi:10.1037/abn0000033

Shorter, E. (2005). *A Historical Dictionary of Psychiatry*, New York, Oxford University Press.

Siever, L. J. & Davis, K. L. (1991). A psychobiological perspective on the personality disorders. *American Journal of Psychiatry*, 148(12),1647–58. doi:10.1176/ajp.148.12.1647

Silberman, E., Balon, R., Starcevic, V., et al. (2020). Benzodiazepines: it's time to return to the evidence. *British Journal of Psychiatry*, 1–3. doi:10.1192/bjp.2020.164

Silk, K. R. & Feurino, L., III. (2012). Psychopharmacology of personality disorders. In Widiger, T. A. (ed.) *The Oxford Handbook of Personality Disorders*. New York, Oxford University Press.

Simon, K. M. (2015). Obsessive–compulsive personality disorder. In Beck, A. T., Davis, D. D. & Freeman, A. (eds.) *Cognitive Therapy of Personality Disorders*. 3rd ed. New York, Guilford Press.

Simonsen, E. & Newton-Howes, G. (2018). Personality pathology and schizophrenia. *Schizophrenia Bulletin*, 44(6),1180–4. doi:10.1093/schbul/sby053

Sinclair, M. & Beadman, M. (2016). *The Little ACT Workbook*, Bath, Crimson Publishing.

Sisti, D., Young, M. & Caplan, A. (2013). Defining mental illnesses: Can values and objectivity get along? *BMC Psychiatry*, 13 (1),346. doi:10.1186/1471-244X-13-346

Skodol, A. E., Gunderson, J. G., McGlashan, T. H., et al. (2002). Functional impairment in patients with schizotypal, borderline, avoidant, or obsessive-compulsive personality disorder. *American Journal of Psychiatry*, 159(2),276–83. doi:10.1176/appi.ajp.159.2.276

Skodol, A. E., Johnson, J. G., Cohen, P., Sneed, J. R. & Crawford, T. N. (2007). Personality disorder and impaired functioning from adolescence to adulthood. *British Journal of Psychiatry* 190(5),415–20. doi:10.1192/bjp.bp.105.019364

Smith, T. E. & Samuel, D. B. (2017). A multi-method examination of the links between ADHD and personality disorder. *Journal of Personality Disorders*, 31(1),26–48. doi:10.1521/pedi_2016_30_236

Soeteman, D. I., Hakkaart-Van Roijen, L., Verheul, R. & Busschbach, J. J. (2008). The economic burden of personality disorders in mental health care. *Journal of Clinical Psychiatry*, 69(2),259–65. doi:10.4088/jcp.v69n0212

Soloff, P. H. (1998). Algorithms for pharmacological treatment of personality dimensions: Symptom-specific treatments for cognitive-perceptual, affective, and impulsive-behavioral dysregulation. *Bulletin of the Menninger Clinic*, 62(2),195–214.

Somma, A., Gialdi, G. & Fossati, A. (2019). Reliability and construct validity of the Personality Inventory for ICD-11 (PiCD) in Italian adult participants. *Psychological Assessment*. doi:10.1037/pas0000766

Spiegel, D. & Kato, P. M. (1996). Psychosocial Influences on cancer incidence and progression. *Harvard Review of Psychiatry*, 4 (1),10–26. doi:10.3109/10673229609030518

Spitzer, R. L., Endicott, J. & Gibbon, M. (1979). Crossing the border into borderline personality and borderline schizophrenia. The development of criteria. *Archives of General Psychiatry*, 36(1),17–24. doi:10.1001/archpsyc.1979.01780010023001

Spitzer, R. L., Williams, J. B. W., Gibbon, M. & First, M. B. (1990). *Structured Clinical Interview for DSM-III-R Personality Disorders (SCID-II)*, Washington, DC, American Psychiatric Association Press.

Stanley, S. H., Laugharne, J. D., Addis, S. & Sherwood, D. (2013). Assessing overweight and obesity across mental disorders: Personality disorders at high risk. *Social Psychiatry and Psychiatric Epidemiology*, 48 (3),487–92. doi:10.1007/s00127-012-0546-1

Stein, G. (2018). *The Hidden Psychiatry of the Old Testament*, Lanham, MD, Hamilton Books (Rowman & Littlefield).

Stephan, Y., Sutin, A. R., Luchetti, M. & Terracciano, A. (2019). Facets of conscientiousness and longevity: Findings from the Health and Retirement Study. *Journal of Psychosomatic Research*, 116, 1–5. doi:10.1016/j.jpsychores.2018.11.002

Stern, B. L., Diamond, D. & Yeomans, F. E. (2017). Transference-focused psychotherapy (TFP) for narcissistic personality: Engaging patients in the early treatment process. *Psychoanalytic Psychology*, 34(4),381–96. doi:10.1037/pap0000145

Stoffers, J. M., Völlm, B. A., Rücker, G., Timmer, A., Huband, N. & Lieb, K. (2012). Psychological therapies for people with borderline personality disorder. *Cochrane Database of Systematic Reviews*, 2012(8), CD005652. doi:10.1002/14651858. CD005652.pub2

Stone, M. H. (2016). Long-term course of borderline personality disorder. *Psychodynamic Psychiatry*, 44(3),449–74. doi:10.1521/pdps.2016.44.3.449

Storebø, O. J., Stoffers-Winterling, J. M., Völlm, B. A., et al. (2020). Psychological therapies for people with borderline personality disorder (Review). *Cochrane Database of Systematic Reviews*, (5), CD012955. doi:10.1002/14651858. CD012955.pub2

Strickhouser, J. E., Zell, E. & Krizan, Z. (2017). Does personality predict health and well-being? A metasynthesis. *Health Psychology*, 36(8),797–810. doi:10.1037/hea0000475

Tattersall, R. B. (1997). Brittle diabetes revisited: The Third Arnold Bloom Memorial Lecture. *Diabetic Medicine*, 14(2),99–110. doi:10.1002/(SICI)1096-9136(199702) 14:2<99::AID-DIA320>3.0.CO;2-I

Taylor, B. (2015). *The Last Asylum: A Memoir of Madness in Our Times*, Chicago, IL, University of Chicago Press.

Teo, A. R. & Gaw, A. C. (2010). Hikikomori, a Japanese culture-bound syndrome of social withdrawal? A proposal for DSM-5. *Journal of Nervous and Mental Disease*, 198(6),444-9. doi:10.1097/NMD.0b013e3181e086b1

Theophrastus (1909). *Theophrastou Charakteres (The Characters of Theophrastus)*, London, Macmillan.

Thornicroft, G. J. (2006). *Actions Speak Louder: Tackling Discrimination against People with Mental Illness*, London, Mental Health Foundation.

Torgersen, S., Kringlen, E. & Cramer, V. (2001). The prevalence of personality disorders in a community sample. *Archives of General Psychiatry*, 58(6),590–6. doi:10.1001/archpsyc.58.6.590

Triandis, H. C. (2001). Individualism-collectivism and personality. *Journal of Personality*, 69(6),907–24. doi:10.1111/1467-6494.696169

Trull, T. J., Jahng, S., Tomko, R. L., Wood, P. K. & Sher, K. J. (2010). Revised NESARC personality disorder diagnoses: Gender, prevalence, and comorbidity with substance dependence disorders. *Journal of Personality Disorders*, 24(4),412–26. doi:10.1521/pedi.2010.24.4.412

Tully, P. J. & Selkow, T. (2014). Personality disorders in heart failure patients requiring psychiatric management: Comorbidity detections from a routine depression and anxiety screening protocol. *Psychiatry Research*, 220(3),954–9. doi:10.1016/j.psychres.2014.08.051

Tyrer, P. (1980). Dependence on benzodiazepines. *British Journal of Psychiatry*, 137(6),576–7. doi:10.1192/bjp.137.6.576

Tyrer, P. (1985). Neurosis divisible? *The Lancet*, 325(8430),685–8. doi:10.1016/s0140-6736(85)91340-6

Tyrer, P. (ed.) (1988). *Personality Disorders: Diagnosis, Management and Course*, London, Wright.

Tyrer, P. (1989). *Classification of Neurosis*, Chichester, John Wiley.

Tyrer, P. (2002). Nidotherapy: A new approach to the treatment of personality disorder. *Acta Psychiatrica Scandinavica*, 105(6),469–71. doi:10.1034/j.1600-0447.2002.01362.x

Tyrer, P. (2009a). *Nidotherapy: Harmonising the Environment with the Patient* (1st ed.), London, RCPsych Publications.

Tyrer, P. (2009b). Why borderline personality disorder is neither borderline nor a personality disorder. *Personality and Mental Health*, 3(2),86–95. doi:10.1002/pmh.78

Tyrer, P. (2012). DSM [100 Words]. *British Journal of Psychiatry*, 200(1),67. doi:10.1192/bjp.bp.111.102970

Tyrer, H. (2013). *Tackling Health Anxiety: A CBT Handbook*, London, RCPsych Publications.

Tyrer, P. (2015). Personality dysfunction is the cause of recurrent non-cognitive mental disorder: A testable hypothesis. *Personality and Mental Health*, 9(1),1–7. doi:10.1002/pmh.1255

Tyrer, P. (2018). Against the Stream: Generalised Anxiety Disorder (GAD) – A redundant diagnosis. *BJPsych Bulletin*, 42 (2),69–71. doi:10.1192/bjb.2017.12

Tyrer, P. (2020a). A national service for personality disorder: A hesitant but important development. *Personality and Mental Health*, 14(3),243–5. doi:10.1002/pmh.1479.

Tyrer, P. (2020b). Personality difficulty. *Revista Latinoamericana de Personalidad*, 1(1),1–3.

Tyrer, P. (2021). *Neurosis: Understanding Common Mental Illness*. Cambridge, Cambridge University Press.

Tyrer, P. & Alexander, J. (1979). Classification of personality disorder. *British Journal of Psychiatry*, 135(2),163–7. doi:10.1192/bjp.135.2.163

Tyrer, P., Alexander, J. & Ferguson, B. (1988). Personality assessment schedule. In Tyrer, P. (ed.) *Personality Disorders: Diagnosis, Management and Course.* London, Wright.

Tyrer, P. & Baldwin, D. (2006). Generalised anxiety disorder. *Lancet* 368(9553),2156–66. doi:10.1016/S0140-6736(06)69865-6

Tyrer, P. & Boardman, J. (2020). Refining social prescribing in the UK. *Lancet Psychiatry*, 7 (10),831–2. doi:10.1016/S2215-0366(20) 30129-2

Tyrer, P., Coombs, N., Ibrahimi, F., et al. (2007). Critical developments in the assessment of personality disorder. *British Journal of Psychiatry*, 190(S49), s51–9. doi:10.1192/bjp.190.5.s51

Tyrer, P., Cooper, S., Rutter, D. et al. (2009). The assessment of dangerous and severe personality disorder: Lessons from a randomised controlled trial linked to qualitative analysis. *Journal of Forensic Psychiatry & Psychology*, 20(1),132–46. doi:10.1080/14789940802236872

Tyrer, P., Cooper, S., Salkovskis, P., et al. (2014a). Clinical and cost-effectiveness of cognitive behaviour therapy for health anxiety in medical patients: A multicentre randomised controlled trial. *The Lancet*, 383 (9913),219–25. doi:10.1016/S0140-6736(13) 61905-4

Tyrer, P., Crawford, M., Mulder, R. T., et al. (2011a). The rationale for the reclassification of personality disorder in the 11th revision of the International Classification of Diseases (ICD-11). *Personality and Mental Health*, 5 (4),246–59. doi:10.1002/pmh.190

Tyrer, P., Crawford, M., Sanatinia, R., et al. (2014b). Preliminary studies of the ICD-11 classification of personality disorder in practice. *Personality and Mental Health*, 8 (4),254–63. doi:10.1002/pmh.1275

Tyrer, P. & Davidson, K. (2000). Cognitive therapy for personality disorders. In Gunderson, J. G. & Gabbard, G. O. (eds.) *Psychotherapy for Personality Disorders.* Washington, DC: American Psychiatric Press.

Tyrer, P., Merson, S., Onyett, S. & Johnson, T. (1994). The effect of personality disorder on clinical outcome, social networks and adjustment: A controlled clinical trial of psychiatric emergencies. *Psychological Medicine*, 24(3),731–40. doi:10.1017/S0033291700027884

Tyrer, P., Milošeska, K., Whittington, C., et al. (2011b). Nidotherapy in the treatment of substance misuse, psychosis and personality disorder: Secondary analysis of a controlled trial. *The Psychiatrist*, 35(1),9–14. doi:10.1192/pb.bp.110.029983

Tyrer, P., Mitchard, S., Methuen, C. & Ranger, M. (2003a). Treatment rejecting and treatment seeking personality disorders: Type R and Type S. *Journal of Personality Disorders*, 17(3),263–8. doi:10.1521/ pedi.17.3.263.22152

Tyrer, P., Morgan, J. & Cicchetti, D. (2004a). The Dependent Personality Questionnaire (DPQ): A screening instrument for dependent personality. *International Journal of Social Psychiatry*, 50(1),10–17. doi:10.1177/0020764004038754

Tyrer, P. & Mulder, R. T. (2018). Dissecting the elements of borderline personality disorder. *Personality and Mental Health*, 12(2),91–2. doi:10.1002/pmh.1422

Tyrer, P., Owen, R. & Dawling, S. (1983). Gradual withdrawal of diazepam after long-term therapy. *Lancet*, 1(8339),1402–6. doi:10.1016/s0140-6736(83)92355-3

Tyrer, P., Reed, G. M. & Crawford, M. J. (2015). Classification, assessment, prevalence, and effect of personality disorder. *Lancet*, 385 (9969),717–26. doi:10.1016/S0140-6736(14) 61995-4

Tyrer, P., Rutherford, D. & Huggett, T. (1981). Benzodiazepine withdrawal symptoms and propranolol. *Lancet* 1(8219),520–2. doi:10.1016/s0140-6736(81)92861-0

Tyrer, P., Seivewright, H. & Johnson, T. (2004b). The Nottingham Study of Neurotic Disorder: Predictors of 12-year outcome of dysthymic, panic and generalized anxiety disorder. *Psychological Medicine*, 34(8),1385–94. doi:10.1017/s0033291704002569

Tyrer, P., Seivewright, N., Ferguson, B., et al. (1990). The Nottingham Study of Neurotic Disorder: Relationship between personality status and symptoms. *Psychological Medicine*, 20(2),423–31. doi:10.1017/ s0033291700017736

Tyrer, P., Seivewright, N., Ferguson, B. & Tyrer, J. (1992). The general neurotic syndrome: A coaxial diagnosis of anxiety, depression and personality disorder. *Acta Psychiatrica Scandinavica*, 85(3),201–6. doi:10.1111/j.1600-0447.1992.tb08595.x

Tyrer, P., Sensky, T. & Mitchard, S. (2003b). Principles of nidotherapy in the treatment of persistent mental and personality disorders. *Psychotherapy and Psychosomatics*, 72 (6),350–6. doi:10.1159/000073032

Tyrer, P., Turner, R. & Johnson, A. L. (1989). Integrated hospital and community psychiatric services and use of inpatient beds. *British Medical Journal (Clinical Research Ed.)*, 299(6694),298–300. doi:10.1136/ bmj.299.6694.298

Tyrer, P. & Tyrer, H. (2018). *Nidotherapy: Harmonising the Environment with the Patient* (2nd ed.), Cambridge, Cambridge University Press/Royal College of Psychiatrists.

Tyrer, P., Tyrer, H. & Guo, B. (2016a). The general neurotic syndrome: A re-evaluation [Editorial]. *Psychotherapy and Psychosomatics*, 85(4),193–7. doi:10.1159/ 000444196.

Tyrer, P., Tyrer, H., Yang, M. & Guo, B. (2016b). Long-term impact of temporary and persistent personality disorder on anxiety and depressive disorders. *Personality and Mental Health*, 10(2),76–83. doi:10.1002/pmh.1324

Tyrer, P., Wang, D., Tyrer, H., et al. (2021). Influence of apparently negative personality characteristics on the long-term outcome of health anxiety: Secondary analysis of a randomized controlled trial. *Personality and Mental Health*, 15(1),72–86. doi:10.1002/ pmh.1496

Tyrer, P., Yang, M. Tyrer, H., & Crawford, M. (2021). Is social function a good proxy measure of personality disorder? . *Personality and Mental Health*, 1–12. https://doi.org/10 .1002/pmh.1513

Van Bronswijk, S. C., Köster, E. M. & Peeters, F. P. M. L. (2020). Effectiveness of acute-phase treatment of depression is not influenced by comorbid personality disorders: Results from a meta-analysis and meta-regression. *Psychotherapy and Psychosomatics*, 89, 109–10. doi:10.1159/ 000502918

Van Heck, G. L. (1997). Personality and physical health: Toward an ecological approach to health-related personality research. *European Journal of Personality*, 11(5),415–43. doi:10.1002/(SICI)1099-0984(199712)11:5<415::AID-PER306>3.0.CO;2-G

Van, H. L. & Kool, M. (2018). What we do, do not, and need to know about comorbid depression and personality disorders. *Lancet Psychiatry*, 5(10),776–8. doi:10.1016/S2215-0366(18)30260-8

Venables, N. C., Hall, J. R. & Patrick, C. J. (2014). Differentiating psychopathy from antisocial personality disorder: A triarchic model perspective. *Psychological Medicine*, 44 (5),1005–13. doi:10.1017/s003329171300161x

Verheul, R., Kranzler, H. R., Poling, J., Tennen, H., Ball, S. & Rounsaville, B. J. (2000). Axis I and Axis II disorders in alcoholics and drug addicts: Fact or artifact? *Journal of Studies on Alcohol*, 61(1),101–10. doi:10.15288/jsa.2000.61.101

Verheul, R. & Widiger, T. A. (2004). A meta-analysis of the prevalence and usage of the personality disorder not otherwise specified (PDNOS) diagnosis. *Journal of Personality Disorders*, 18(4),309–19. doi:10.1521/pedi.18.4.309.40350

Viding, E. (2019). *Psychopathy: A very short introduction*, New York, Oxford University Press.

Viding, E., Blair, R. J., Moffitt, T. E. & Plomin, R. (2005). Evidence for substantial genetic risk for psychopathy in 7-year-olds. *Journal of Child Psychology and Psychiatry*, 46(6),592–7. doi:10.1111/j.1469-7610.2004.00393.x

Volkert, J., Gablonski, T. C. & Rabung, S. (2018). Prevalence of personality disorders in the general adult population in Western countries: Systematic review and meta-analysis. *British Journal of Psychiatry*, 213(6),709–15. doi:10.1192/bjp.2018.202

Wachtel, P. L. (1973). Psychodynamics, behavior therapy, and the implacable experimenter: An inquiry into the consistency of personality. *Journal of Abnormal Psychology*, 82(2),324–34. doi:10.1037/h0035132

Watters, E. (2010). The Americanization of Mental Illness. *New York Times*, Jan 8, p. MM40.

Weekers, L. C., Hutsebaut, J. & Kamphuis, J. H. (2019). The Level of Personality Functioning Scale-Brief Form 2.0: Update of a brief instrument for assessing level of personality functioning. *Personality and Mental Health*, 13(1),3–14. doi:10.1002/pmh.1434

Weiner, H., Reiser, M. F., Thaler, M. & Mirsky, I. A. (1957). Etiology of duodenal ulcer: I. Relation of specific psychological characteristics to rate of gastric secretion (serum pepsinogen) [Special article/Book review]. *Psychosomatic Medicine*, 19 (1),1–10. doi:10.1097/00006842-195701000-00001

Widiger, T. A., De Clercq, B. & De Fruyt, F. (2009). Childhood antecedents of personality disorder: An alternative perspective. *Development and Psychopathology*, 21 (3),771–91. doi:10.1017/S095457940900042X

Widiger, T. A. & Oltmanns, J. R. (2016). The ICD-11 proposals and field trials. *Personality and Mental Health*, 10(2),120–2. doi:10.1002/pmh.1341

Widiger, T. A. & Trull, T. J. (1992). Personality and psychopathology: An application of the Five-Factor Model. *Journal of Personality*, 60 (2),363–93. doi:10.1111/j.1467-6494.1992.tb00977.x

Williams, P. & Balestrieri, M. (1989). Psychiatric clinics in general practice: Do they reduce admissions? *British Journal of Psychiatry*, 154 (1),67–71. doi:10.1192/bjp.154.1.67

Winokur, G., Behar, D., Van Valkenburg, C. & Lowry, M. (1978). Is a familial definition of depression both feasible and valid? *Journal of Nervous & Mental Disease*, 166(11),764–8. doi:10.1097/00005053-197811000-00002

Winsper, C., Bilgin, A., Thompson, A., Marwaha, S., et al. (2020). The prevalence of personality disorders in the community: A global systematic review and meta-analysis. *British Journal of Psychiatry*, 216(2),69–78. doi:10.1192/bjp.2019.166

Wolpert, L. (2001). Stigma of depression–a personal view. *British Medical Bulletin*, 57 (1),221–4. doi:10.1093/bmb/57.1.221

World Health Organization (1992). *The ICD-10 Classification of Mental and Behavioural Disorders: Diagnostic Criteria for Research*, Geneva, WHO.

World Health Organization. (2018). *ICD-11, the 11th Revision of the International Classification of Diseases* [Online]. Geneva: World Health Organization. Available: https://icd.who.int/ [Accessed 21 January 2021].

Yang, M., Coid, J. & Tyrer, P. (2010). Personality pathology recorded by severity: National survey. *British Journal of Psychiatry*, 197 (3),193–9. doi:10.1192/bjp.bp.110.078956

Yang, M., Tyrer H., Johnson T. & Tyrer P. (2021). Personality change in the Nottingham Study of Neurotic Disorder: 30 year cohort study. *Australian and New Zealand Journal of Psychiatry*, Jul 10:48674211025624. doi: 10.1177/00048674211025624. Online ahead of print

Yen, S., Shea, M. T., Battle, C. L., et al. (2002). Traumatic exposure and posttraumatic stress disorder in borderline, schizotypal, avoidant, and obsessive-compulsive personality disorders: Findings from the collaborative longitudinal personality disorders study. *Journal of Nervous and Mental Disease*, 190 (8),510–18. doi:10.1097/00005053-200208000-00003

Yeomans, F. (2007). Questions concerning the randomized trial of schema-focused therapy vs transference-focused psychotherapy. *Archives of General Psychiatry*, 64(5),609–11. doi:10.1001/archpsyc.64.5.609-c

Yoshimasu, K., Barbaresi, W. J., Colligan, R. C., et al. (2012). Childhood ADHD is strongly associated with a broad range of psychiatric disorders during adolescence: A population-based birth cohort study. *Journal of Child Psychology and Psychiatry*, 53 (10),1036–43. doi:10.1111/j.1469-7610.2012.02567.x

Zanarini, M. C., Frankenburg, F. R., Hennen, J. & Silk, K. R. (2003). The longitudinal course of borderline psychopathology: 6-year prospective follow-up of the phenomenology of borderline personality disorder. *American Journal of Psychiatry*, 160(2),274–283. doi:10.1176/appi.ajp.160.2.274

Zanarini, M. C., Frankenburg, F. R., Reich, D. B., Conkey, L. C. & Fitzmaurice, G. M. (2015). Treatment rates for patients with borderline personality disorder and other personality disorders: A 16-year study. *Psychiatric Services* 66(1),15–20. doi:10.1176/appi.ps.201400055

Zanarini, M. C., Frankenburg, F. R., Reich, D. B. & Fitzmaurice, G. (2012a). Attainment and stability of sustained symptomatic remission and recovery among patients with borderline personality disorder and axis II comparison subjects: A 16-year prospective follow-up study. *American Journal of Psychiatry*, 169 (5),476–83. doi:10.1176/appi.ajp.2011.11101550

Zanarini, M. C., Hörz-Sagstetter, S., Temes, C. M., et al. (2019). The 24-year course of major depression in patients with borderline personality disorder and personality-disordered comparison subjects. *Journal of Affective Disorders*, 258, 109–14. doi:10.1016/j.jad.2019.08.005

Zanarini, M. C., Schulz, S. C., Detke, H., et al. (2012b). Open-label treatment with olanzapine for patients with borderline personality disorder. *Journal of Clinical Psychopharmacology*, 32(3),398–402. doi:10.1097/JCP.0b013e3182524293

Zettle, R. D. (2003). Acceptance and Commitment Therapy (ACT) vs. systematic desensitization in treatment of mathematics anxiety. *The Psychological Record*, 53 (2),197–215. doi:10.1007/BF03395440

Zimmerman, M. (1994). Diagnosing personality disorders. A review of issues and research methods. *Archives of General Psychiatry*, 51 (3),225–45. doi:10.1001/archpsyc.1994.03950030061006

INDEX